Accelerated Education in Nursing

Lin Zhan, PhD, RN, FAAN, received a PhD from Boston College, a Master of Science from Boston University, and a Bachelor of Science from West China University of Medical Sciences. Currently, Dr. Zhan is a Dean and Professor, Loewenberg School of Nursing, University of Memphis.

Zhan is a Fellow of American Academy of Nursing (FAAN). Her program of research focuses on quality of life of older adults and ethnic minorities, and her scholarly work is evident by funded research projects. Dr. Zhan was a Research Fellow at Boston's Hebrew Rehabilitation Center for Aged where she studied family caregiving for persons with Alzheimer's disease under the NIH K24 Grant. She has published near 100 articles and five edited books, and delivered keynotes and speeches nationally and internationally.

Dr. Zhan is on the American Academy of Nursing Expert Panel on Aging, an Associate in the Institute for Nursing Healthcare Leadership, Boston, a Clinical Scientist at Phyllis F. Cantor Center for Research, Dana-Farber Cancer Institute, and has served on the Board of Governors of National League for Nursing in New York. Internationally, Zhan is a visiting/honorary professor in 10 of the Chinese universities, and served as a consultant for Partner Harvard Medical International (2008–2010).

Zhan has received numerous regional, national, and international awards for her excellence in education, service, scholarship, and leadership.

Linda P. Finch, PhD, RN, APN, received a PhD from the University of Memphis, a Master of Nursing Science degree from the University of Arkansas for Medical Sciences, a Bachelor of Science in Nursing degree from Memphis State University, and a nursing diploma from Baptist Memorial Hospital School of Nursing. Dr. Finch is Associate Dean and Associate Professor, Loewenberg School of Nursing, at the University of Memphis. She is a board certified Adult Nurse Practitioner.

Dr. Finch's program of research focuses on communication and caring, particularly the nurse–patient relationship and patient outcomes. In addition to identifying behavioral markers of nurse caring, her work generated a substantive theory of nurse caring; Personalized Nurse Caring.

Dr. Finch has numerous peer-reviewed publications and presentations at state, national, and international conferences. Finch is a member of Sigma Theta Tau International (STTI) Nursing Honor Society, the American Nurses' Association (ANA), is an ANA Dorothy Cornelius Scholar, and is a Fellow in the Leadership for Academic Nursing Program sponsored by the American Association of Colleges of Nursing. Finch is a reviewer for the *Journal of Nursing Scholarship*, STTI, and is on the editorial board of the *Tennessee Nurse*.

Accelerated Education in Nursing

Challenges, Strategies, and Future Directions

Lin Zhan, PhD, RN, FAAN

Linda P. Finch, PhD, RN, APN

Editors

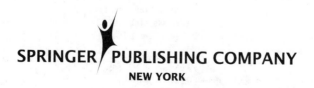

SPRINGER PUBLISHING COMPANY

NEW YORK

Springer Publishing Company, LLC
11 West 42nd Street
New York, NY 10036
www.springerpub.com

Acquisitions Editor: Allan Graubard
Composition: Techset

ISBN: 978-0-8261-0763-3
E-book ISBN: 978-0-8261-0764-0

11 12 13/ 5 4 3 2 1

The author and the publisher of this Work have made every effort to use sources believed to be reliable to provide information that is accurate and compatible with the standards generally accepted at the time of publication. The author and publisher shall not be liable for any special, consequential, or exemplary damages resulting, in whole or in part, from the readers' use of, or reliance on, the information contained in this book. The publisher has no responsibility for the persistence or accuracy of URLs for external or third-party Internet Web sites referred to in this publication and does not guarantee that any content on such Web sites is, or will remain, accurate or appropriate.

Library of Congress Cataloging-in-Publication Data

CIP data is available at the Library of Congress

Printed in the United States of America by Bang Printing

*This book is dedicated to our families
for their continuing love and support.*

Lin Zhan and Linda P. Finch

Contents

Contributors

Geraldine Polly Bednash, PhD, RN, FAAN, Chief Executive Officer and Executive Director, American Association of Colleges of Nursing, Washington, DC

Susan B. Belinsky, EdD, RT (R) (CT), Director, Radiation Therapy Program, School of Medical Imaging and Therapeutics, Massachusetts College of Pharmacy and Health Sciences, Boston, MA

Melissa R. Boellaard, MSN, RN, Clinical Instructor, Department of Nursing, College of Nursing and Health Sciences, University of Wisconsin-Eau Claire, Eau Claire, WI

Cheryl L. Brandt, PhD, ACNS-BC, Associate Professor, Department of Nursing, College of Nursing and Health Sciences, University of Wisconsin-Eau Claire, Eau Claire, WI

Linda M. Caldwell, DNSc, ANP-BC, Curry College, Division of Nursing, Milton, MA

Jill Dapremont, EdD, RN, Assistant Professor, Loewenberg School of Nursing, The University of Memphis, Memphis, TN

Vernell P. DeWitty, PhD, RN, Program Deputy Director, Robert Wood Johnson New Careers in Nursing, American Association of Colleges of Nursing, Washington, DC

Di Fang, PhD, Director of Research and Data Services, American Association of Colleges of Nursing, Washington, DC

Lisa Fanning, MEd, RT (R) (CT), Director of Radiography, School of Medical Imaging and Therapeutics, Massachusetts College of Pharmacy and Health Sciences, Weymouth, MA

Janet Fraser Hale, PhD, RN, FNP, Associate Dean for Academic Affairs, Director of Interprofessional and Community Partnerships, Graduate School of Nursing, University of Massachusetts Medical School, Worcester, MA

Alicia Huckstadt, PhD, ARNP-FNP-BC, Professor & Director of Graduate Nursing Program, Wichita State University, Wichita, KS

Terri Jabaley, PhD, RN, PhD candidate, Assistant Professor, Department of Nursing, Emmanuel College, Boston, MA

Mahmoud Kaddoura, PhD, CAGS, MED, MSN, BSN, RN, Assistant Professor, Massachusetts College of Pharmacy and Health Sciences, Boston, MA

Frances K. Keech, RT (N), MBA, FSNMTS, Associate Professor, Nuclear Medicine Technology Program Director, Boston, MA

Michael Kneeland, MD, Associate Dean of Allied Health and Interprofessional Education, University of Massachusetts Medical School, Worcester, MA

Susan A. LaRocco, PhD, RN, MBA, Professor, Curry College Milton, Charlestown, MA

Shirleatha Lee, PhD, RN, CNE, Assistant Professor, Loewenberg School of Nursing, The University of Memphis, Memphis, TN

Michele Pugnaire, MD, Senior Associate Dean, Educational Affairs, University of Massachusetts Medical School, Worchester, MA

Kathy Ride-Out, EdD, PNP-BC, FNAP, Senior Associate Dean for Academic Affairs, University of Rochester School of Nursing, Rochester, NY

Paulette Seymour-Route, PhD, RN, Dean and Professor, Graduate School of Nursing, University of Massachusetts, Worcester, MA

David M. M. Sharp, MA (Hons), RMN, RGN, MSc (Nurse Education), RNT, PhD, MSc (Social Anth) RN, Professor of Nursing, School of Nursing and Allied Health, Louisiana College School of Nursing, Pineville, LA

Kimberly J. Sharp, BA, BSc, RN, MSc (Nurse Education), OHND, PhD, Dean, School of Nursing and Allied Health, Louisiana College, Pineville, LA

Collette Williams, RN, MSN, PhD (C), Clinical Education Manager, Quincy Hospital, Boston, MA

CeCelia R. Zorn, PhD, RN, Professor, Department of Nursing, College of Nursing and Health Sciences, University of Wisconsin-Eau Claire, Eau Claire, WI

Foreword

Nurse educators have a long tradition of creative development in nursing education programs. The vast array of program types for individuals with various levels of nursing education have been a direct response of the awareness by nurse educators that multiple streams of learning can result in very high-quality educational outcomes. Thus, deans of nursing in baccalaureate and higher-degree programs have designed programs that take into account the education previously acquired by learners. Review of reports from schools of nursing provide evidence of these non-traditional educational pathways with multiple institutions offering programs such as LPN to BSN, ADN to MSN, and/or fast track to the PhD.

These innovative programs are also a direct result of clear indications that a pool of potential students, interested in advancing their education in nursing, will enroll and take advantage of their creative programs to improve their capacity to deliver high-quality nursing care. In the last two decades, a different pool of potential students have shaped nursing education in a markedly different and creative way. These students, termed as second-degree or second-career students, are stimulated to seek a career in nursing as a result of policy makers' and health care organizations' clear message to the public that professional nurses are paramount to the delivery of high quality health care to diverse populations. Another positive impetus for these students to pursue a nursing degree is the rewards associated with a career as a professional nurse. Consequently, the response of second-career/-degree students is overwhelmingly positive as they seek out programs that will prepare them for a career in nursing.

As will be described in this important book—*Accelerated Education in Nursing: Challenges, Strategies, and Future Directions*—the result has been the development of programs that are designed to recognize the previous academic experiences of the second-career/second-degree students and assure as rapid completion of the nursing curriculum as possible while sustaining quality and integrity of accelerated nursing programming. While accelerated degree programs vary in length, all focus on an intensification and compression of the nursing course work that facilitates rapid completion. Student learners experience the nursing curriculum with full-time study and daily experiences complete with intense clinical exposures to the practice of professional nursing. A sign of these programs' success is the strong employer acceptance for the graduates who are committed nursing professionals with a wealth of experience to bring to their nursing practice.

Accelerated degree programs provide evidence that creativity in nursing program design can facilitate learning experiences that assure competence in the profession while also taking advantage of the knowledge, skills, and experiences the learner brings to our profession. Lessons learned from accelerated nursing programs can be applied in all our programs and enrich the education of professional nurses, who are essential in meeting the health care needs of the public.

Geraldine Polly Bednash, PhD, RN, FAAN
CEO, AACN

Preface

Accelerated programs in nursing have gained popularity over the last 10 years in responding to a shortage of baccalaureate-prepared nurses, accommodating learning needs of a special pool of learners with prior university/college education, and meeting the need for advanced practice nurses and educators. A handful of accelerated nursing programs directly enroll high-school graduates and provide the baccalaureate degree within a 32-month college educational framework. Concomitantly, there is a growing concern in the public about the safety and quality of patients seeking health care services, thus, increasing an oversight for readiness and competencies of new nursing graduates for contemporary practice.

Does accelerated nursing education prepare graduates with essential knowledge and critical skills for contemporary practice? Does the accelerated nursing education model provide a substantive, sustained, and innovative approach to nursing in curriculum reform? What challenges do faculty, students, and administrators face in accelerated nursing education? What strategies are used to sustain and improve quality and integrity of accelerated nursing education? To date, a paucity of literature exists that explores, describes, and examines critical issues in accelerated nursing education. It is with this intent, therefore, that this book, *Accelerated Nursing Education: Challenges, Strategies, and Future Directions* (hereafter, the book), is written by and for nursing faculty, health professionals, researchers, and academic leaders.

The book is organized into three sections. Section I: Achieving Excellence in Accelerated Nursing Education is composed of six chapters that focus on description and examination of curriculum innovation, student learning, faculty teaching, and workable strategies to achieve excellence in accelerated nursing education. In Chapter 1: Accelerated Nursing Education: An Overview, Dr. Finch examines accelerated nursing education from historical, social, and higher-education perspectives. Although the current literature on accelerated nursing education is limited, this chapter provides an overview of students' demographic characteristics, program retention and outcome issues, and effective faculty teaching. Issues and challenges for accelerated nursing program faculty and students are presented, along with the need to continue research that examines effectiveness of accelerated nursing programs.

Dr. Kaddoura and associates present Chapter 2: Curriculum Innovation. This chapter provides a review of current literature in curriculum innovation and models of using knowledge to create new ways (contents, pedagogy, and experience) of teaching. The authors describe challenges faced and strategies used to design and implement innovative curriculum in accelerated nursing programs, and share their experiences about how to manage essential contents, understand student diversity and learning patterns, and integrate active learning methods in classroom and clinical settings. The authors suggest that clinical partnerships, integrated curriculum, coaching, and student-centered, active-learning strategies be used to promote students' learning.

What is an innovative approach to accelerated students' clinical learning? In Chapter 3: Clinical Immersion as an Innovative Pedagogical Approach in Accelerated BSN Programs, Dr. Kaddoura and associates discuss a Clinical Immersion Model (CIM) used in the accelerated BSN program. The CIM allows accelerated students to be immersed in clinical experience after extensive exposure to the theoretical component of nursing courses, which changes the traditional clinical rotation model. The CIM shows promise in making more meaningful connections between didactic and clinical education, and promoting students' clinical thinking and reasoning. Faculty partner with clinical nurses and rethink their roles and expectations.

What constitutes effectiveness of teaching in accelerated nursing education? In Chapter 4: Achieving Excellence in Teaching, Dr. Huckstadt explores issues, strategies, and successes of using evidence-based teaching practice in accelerated nursing education. Teaching effectiveness is a complex and multifactorial concept that involves the teaching–learning dynamics between faculty and students and assessment of students' learning outcomes. The majority of current nursing baccalaureate students are considered "millennial learners," born between 1980 and 2000, technologically adept, and multitaskers. Workable teaching strategies enhance learning outcomes of accelerated students, such as incorporating their previous college experiences and using a wide variety of teaching and learning methods. To achieve excellence in teaching, faculty analyze feedback from a variety of resources to improve effectiveness, adjust teaching methods according to diverse needs of learners, evaluate teaching effectiveness using valid and reliable instruments, and mentor novice educators to the academic role.

Moreover, higher education is held accountable for students' learning outcomes: retention, graduation, and achievement. In Chapter 5: Recruitment, Retention, and Success in Accelerated Baccalaureate Nursing Programs, Drs. Sharp and Sharp analyze a multifaceted phenomenon of accelerated students and discuss challenges and strategies to achieve student retention, progression, and success. Marketing, admission protocol, interviews, cohort viability, and students' motivation are considered factors for recruitment. Accelerated students respond well to a learner-centered teaching approach, where they take the initiative in their learning experience through strategies such as reflective journals, group work, and problem- focused learning. An accelerated program of study does not equal an abbreviated program, and thus, special efforts are made to understand accelerated students, help them to manage stress, and transition them into an accelerated program and ultimately into the nursing profession. Drs. Sharp and Sharp assert that tailored interventions are needed to help disadvantaged students in the accelerated program.

What are the experiences of nursing faculty in accelerated nursing programs? Dr. Brandt and associates share their stories in Chapter 6: The Faculty Experience: Thriving in the Midst of Intensity While Pursuing Excellence. As faculty members teaching accelerated students, their lived experiences reflect their dedication and determination to shape one mind at a time and to cultivate students' critical reasoning in dynamic and complex clinical settings. Faculty stories show their commitment to practicing core values of caring, compassion, and humanity in the dynamic processes of teaching and learning. "Ah-ha moments" experienced by accelerated students, in the authors' own words, are "*the beauty and the beast of the nursing profession*" in which nurse educators make meaningful connections between "ideal" and "real" health care settings. These faculty stories are telling, and in the midst of the fast-paced accelerated program, we discover the essence of faculty excellence.

Section 2: Leadership in Accelerated Nursing Education focuses on the need for leadership to achieve academic excellence and discusses leadership challenges in accelerated nursing programs. What are the leadership challenges? How do academic leaders face these challenges? These questions are addressed in this section, comprising four chapters. In Chapter 7: Leading and Inspiring a Shared Vision, Drs. Lee and Dapremont discuss how academic leaders lead and inspire a shared vision to achieve excellence in accelerated nursing education. Transformative leadership is advocated as it engages, empowers, and enables faculty. It is essential for faculty involvement in decision making related to designing and implementing an accelerated nursing program. Leading requires open communication, transparency, honesty, and integrity. Leaders prepare for challenges that may arise during or after development of the vision, and a shared vision energizes, motivates, and inspires collective processes toward successful outcomes.

As accelerated nursing programs are growing, a critical question is asked, "How do we ensure high quality and integrity of these programs?" Nursing education is held accountable and responsible to prepare graduates for competently entering the nursing profession and/or effectively assuming leadership roles in health care settings. In Chapter 8: Continuous Quality Improvement: Achieving Excellence, Dr. Zhan asserts a practice of continuous quality improvement (CQI) to facilitate changes and innovations and to improve outcomes. Historical perspectives of CQI in the business world and health care sectors are examined. Quality improvement is defined and major principles are examined. Using CQI to achieve excellence is discussed in the context of accelerated nursing students, faculty, and curriculum. The author suggests that academic leaders be committed to creating a culture that embraces quality improvement, building a team that shares common understanding of systems and processes for quality improvement, using a strategic plan that serves as a roadmap for actions, and managing by facts that use data to aid decision making.

Nursing is experiencing an unprecedented shortage of faculty with a terminal degree. Academic leaders are challenged to develop mechanisms and strategies for successful recruitment, retention, and development of nursing faculty. In Chapter 9: Current and Future Needs of Accelerated Nursing Programs: Faculty Recruitment, Retention, and Development, Dr. Rideout examines strategies in faculty recruitment (e.g., collaborative affiliations), faculty retention (e.g., mentoring), and faculty development (e.g., tailored interventions). Development of faculty from a novice to an expert is a continuous process. As faculty are supported and developed, they bring the best practices to teaching future nurses, leaders, and nurse scientists.

Creating and sustaining an accelerated nursing program involves making critical decisions about necessary educational resources needed to support teaching, learning, and fulfilling the institution's mission. The current economic downturn has taken a toll on higher education, resulting in increased student tuition and fees, budget cuts, and/or layoffs of staff. Nurse educators and leaders must be business savvy to meet educational demands for preparing the needed nursing workforce while finding cost-effective ways to sustain the nursing program. Consideration must also be given to professional program accreditation requirements and adequate resources in support of nursing educational programs.

Drs. Caldwell and LaRocco, in Chapter 10: Educational Resources for Accelerated Nursing Programs: Challenges, Strategies, and Future Directions, suggest ways to maximize education resources, including academic and practice-setting collaborations, efficient staffing and scheduling, and use of technology. Essentially, well-thought-out assessment and planning help in balancing demands and supplies, and ultimately, ensure effective allocation and use of resources.

Accelerated programs are developed in response to the demands of the health care workforce. In addition to nursing, there is a shortage of allied health professionals, and as a result, accelerated educational programs in allied health are also growing. Are there differences and/or similarities between allied health and nursing accelerated programs? What are the challenges that allied health accelerated programs face? What strategies are used to achieve program excellence? Which strategies from allied health accelerated programs may be useful to enhance nursing accelerated education? Section 3: Accelerated Nursing Education: Interprofessional Approach, begins with Chapter 11: Accelerated Education in Radiologic Sciences: A Broader Perspective. Professor Fanning et al. discuss how to design an accelerated curriculum and share learning experiences, and teach interventions that support student and program success. Differences in European, Australian, and the United States accelerated bachelor degree programs in radiological sciences are examined. Faculty and staff roles and responsibilities are discussed, as the burden of the successful accelerated educational programs rests heavily on the faculty, with support from administrators and institutions, to meet the workforce needs of radiological professionals.

Crossing the Quality Chasm by the Institute of Medicine (2001) documents disturbing shortfalls in the quality of health care in the United States, and recommends that health professionals deliver patient-centered care as members of an interdisciplinary team. In Chapter 12: Interprofessional Education: The Role of Accelerated Nursing Programs in Preparing the Nurse of the Future, Drs. Seymour-Route and Hale examine models of interprofessional education and its significant implications for preparing nurses in an environment where interprofessional teamwork, communication, and collaboration are valued and taught. Evidence shows that team-based and coordinated care provides the best approach to providing safe, high-quality, patient care. Authors analyze challenges to interprofessional education: disciplinary silos, reward and recognition processes, students, resources, and promotion and tenure. Exemplars of current and future interprofessional initiatives are presented. The authors call for embracing changes to prepare contemporary practitioners who ultimately bring the best outcome for promoting health for patients and diverse populations.

While the first accelerated baccalaureate program for nonnursing college graduates was introduced at St. Louis University in 1971, the American Association of Colleges of Nursing first reported data on numbers and types of accelerated nursing programs in 1990 and 1994. Even to date there are no published data that provide for in-depth analysis of accelerated programs over time. In Chapter 13: The Growth of Accelerated BSN and MSN programs in the United States: A National Perspective, Drs. Fang, Bednash, and DeWitty document the historical growth of the accelerated program, growth variations, demographic characteristics of students in the second-degree programs, and projected future growth of second-degree BSN programs. Continuing expansion of accelerated nursing education needs further research that generates knowledge and strategies to bring the best learning outcomes to nursing students.

The book reflects the collective wisdom and insights borne from the rich experiences of faculty, researchers, and academic administrators who design, implement, research, and evaluate accelerated programs. The central themes of the book are: innovative curriculum; student-centered teaching and clinical learning; faculty experiences in achieving excellence; leadership commitment to quality and integrity of accelerated education; and innovative educational models that are necessary to help prepare future health care practitioners who are caring, compassionate, and competent to promote health and improve patient care outcomes. Still, questions remain to be answered: "What, in the long run, are the pros and cons for moving through nursing education and into the workforce at such a brisk pace?" "Does the fast-paced program deprive students of their time to roam intellectually, grow up, and engage in extracurricular activities?" It may be more palatable to conduct rigorous research that provides evidence to aid decision making and that informs higher-education policy. Nevertheless, accelerated nursing education shows promising outcomes as described in this book.

Accelerated education, like colleges and universities, is seen as an engine of economic and social development. Indeed, accelerated education is a forum for academic freedom, innovation, and rigor that sustains intellectual diversity and vitality in response to changing societal needs. Accelerated nursing education allows faculty, students, and leaders to collaboratively build a vision and face challenges in higher education.

—*Lin Zhan, PhD, RN, FAAN*
—*Linda P. Finch, PhD, RN, APN*

REFERENCE

Institute of Medicine, Committee on Quality Health Care in America. (2001). *Crossing the Quality Chasm: A New Health System for the 21st Century.* Washington, DC: National Academies Press.

Acknowledgments

We would like to acknowledge all contributing authors—*educators, researchers, and/or academic leaders*—who generously commit their time and intellects by sharing their experience, sometime struggles, expertise, and knowledge in building, sustaining, and advancing accelerated education.

We wish to especially thank Dr. Bednash for her generous and thoughtful comments in the Foreword and Springer Publishing Company for their conviction of the importance of this book in academia.

A special thanks to Everlena Smith and Alfreda Davis, our Administrative Assistants, for their ongoing supportive efforts. Without the generous help of all these individuals, this book would not have been possible.

We are indebted to students and faculty who always remind us about our responsibilities and inspire us to work toward betterment of accelerated education.

—*Lin Zhan, PhD, RN, FAAN*
—*Linda P. Finch, PhD, RN, APN*

Achieving Excellence in Accelerated Nursing Education

Accelerated Nursing Education:
An Overview

Linda P. Finch

OVERVIEW: A HISTORICAL PERSPECTIVE

*N*ursing education historically changes to meet the demands of the public. Specifically over the last 40 years and in recent decades, the nation's increasing elderly population and nursing shortage have created a rising call for more nurses, forcing academic communities to act quickly to create solutions (Ouellet & MacIntosh, 2007). Currently, the Bureau of Labor Statistics (2010) projects that there will be a need for 1 million new and replacement registered nurses by the year 2012 and the need for more than 580,000 new and replacement registered nurses by the year 2018. The challenge is to quickly produce competent nurses while maintaining the academic integrity and reputations of the nursing programs (AACN, 2010).

Owing to the recent economic downturn, there is unprecedented rise in persons experiencing long-term unemployment (Bureau of Labor Statistics, 2011). Many college graduates are unable to find jobs in their fields, making educational opportunities, such as accelerated nursing programs, a viable way to retool for entering a profession that is able to compete in today's job market. While the traditional baccalaureate degree is the entry-to-practice standard for professional nursing, there is a new innovative nursing educational model that offers an accelerated degree for nonnursing graduates (AACN, 2010). "Offered at both the baccalaureate and master's degree levels, these programs build on previous learning experiences and transition individuals with undergraduate degrees in other disciplines into nursing" (AACN, 2010, para. 2).

For students with a previously earned degree, accelerated baccalaureate programs offer the fastest way to become a registered nurse with most programs 12 – 18 months in length. Generic master's degree programs can also be accelerated and are geared to nonnursing graduates. These programs generally take 3 years to finish by completing baccalaureate-level nursing courses the first year and graduate courses during the next 2 years of study (AACN, 2010).

Accelerated nursing programs are mostly geared toward the "no nonsense" student and tap into a previously untapped pool of learners to respond to the unique educational demands of nontraditional students (Ouellet & MacIntosh, 2007). The accelerated programs recruit mature students in search of a second career, who already have a baccalaureate or higher degree in a field other than nursing (Cangelosi & Whitt, 2005). These nontraditional students bring an increased level of maturity and previous life experiences that assist with developing essential critical-thinking and professional decision-making skills (Cangelosi & Whitt, 2005) necessary to acquire the educational competencies, complete the second degree quicker, and be ready to enter the nursing work force (AACN, 2010).

While the first accelerated baccalaureate nursing program in the United States was instituted in 1971 at Saint Louis University and still exists (Saint Louis University School of Nursing Accelerated One-Year BSN: Introduction, n.d., para. 2), these programs have reproduced at a very rapid pace. In 1988 there were 10 programs, and by 1990, 31 accelerated baccalaureate programs (BSN) and 12 generic master's programs (MSN) were offered around the country (AACN, 2010). By 2008, the AACN reported 205 active accelerated programs in the United States, with 37 in the planning stages (Lindsey, 2009). Currently, there are 230 accelerated BSN programs in operation, with 33 new programs in the planning stages (AACN, 2010).

REVIEW OF LITERATURE

Despite dramatic increases in the number of accelerated programs currently in the United States, there is a paucity of published research on accelerated programs. A majority of studies on accelerated nursing programs report findings related to student demographics, effective teaching strategies, and program retention and outcomes.

Student Demographics and Characteristics

Cangelosi and Whitt (2005) conducted a literature review of accelerated nursing programs and found that accelerated students tend to be older, married, and more often male when compared with traditional students. Seldomridge and DiBartolo (2005) profiled second-degree nursing students to determine how they differ from traditional nursing students. They reported that the majority of students were European-American, non-Hispanic women, less than 30 years of age, and returning to college to pursue a second bachelor's degree within 5 years of completing their first degree. The educational backgrounds of second-degree students vary, but biology and psychology degrees are the most prevalent (Seldomridge & DiBartolo, 2005).

Accelerated students are motivated to choose second-degree nursing programs because of perceived enhanced financial stability and more employment opportunities, short program lengths, flexible work hours, and previous positive experiences with nurses (Seldomridge & DiBartolo, 2005). Accelerated students also tend to have higher grade point averages (GPAs) than traditional nursing program students (AACN, 2010).

Penprase and Koczara (2009) describe the type of accelerated nursing students who are successful and explore the implications that these programs have on the nursing community as a whole. Their findings support the AACN descriptions that the typical second-degree nursing student "is motivated, older, and has higher academic expectations than high school-entry baccalaureate students" (AACN, 2010, Changing Gears: Second-Degree Students, para. 1). Furthermore, the accelerated second-degree nursing students are "competitive, maintain high GPAs, and almost always pass the NCLEX-RN on the first attempt" (AACN, 2010, para. 4).

Penprase and Koczara (2009) maintain that it is essential to know the typical student demographics and characteristics of accelerated second-degree students to effectively recruit students for programs. An additional recommendation is to interview applicants prior to admission to identify those who are best suited for an accelerated program.

Effective Teaching Strategies

The study by Walker et al. (2007) highlights the importance of faculty–student relationships and the teaching–learning methodologies preferred by second-degree students compared to traditional students. Their findings indicate second-degree BSN students have stronger predilections in the areas of self-directed learning and motivation, trust that faculty will tell them what they need to know, and greater preference for web-based instruction, case studies, and handouts in comparison with traditional students. In addition, the second-degree BSN students have higher expectations for guidance from faculty, classroom structure, and a desire for faculty to know them by name (Walker et al., 2007). A key expectation of an accelerated program is identifying practices that "help build on previous learning experiences" (Tanner, 2006, p. 99). Teaching strategies like simulations, contemporary topics, interactive technology, and case-based problem-solving benefit an accelerated students' ability to learn (Cangelosi & Whitt, 2005). Therefore, increasing the use of online instruction as well as completing the theory portion of the course the first half of the term and the clinical component the last portion of the term are effective curricular approaches (Lindsey, 2009).

Collaborative teaching models promote communication between and among students and faculty. This model identifies nursing faculty to be specifically assigned to teach only accelerated students in classroom and clinical settings. The collaborative teaching model results indicate increased student and faculty program satisfaction, increased student knowledge in evidence-based practice (EBP), and achievement of more efficient learning experiences, a critical element in accelerated nursing programs (Kruszewski, Brough, & Killeen, 2009).

Program Retention and Outcomes

Accelerated programs provide the opportunity for quick entry into the workforce and provide health care facilities with the opportunity to help ease their nursing shortage (Lindsey, 2009). However, program retention issues for second-degree students include increased attrition for several reasons, including the rapid curriculum pace and intensity, personal issues, financial hardships, and employment during the nursing program (Lindsey). Furthermore, Seldomridge and DiBartolo (2005) note that students withdrew from accelerated second-degree nursing programs because of the rapid pace and program intensity that led to poor academic performance, while other students simply determined that nursing was not what they expected. While Seldomridge and DiBartolo (2005) report that nursing academic performance strongly correlates with success on the NCLEX-RN, there are no significant differences between NCLEX-RN pass rates of traditional versus accelerated students.

In general, accelerated second-degree students are older, mature, highly independent, and motivated learners who benefit from more autonomy and flexibility as well as creative learning within educational programs.

Therefore, it is often the experienced faculty who can implement creative teaching methodologies and offer support to accelerated students essential for meeting their educational demands and expectations.

ISSUES AND CHALLENGES

The growth and development of accelerated nursing programs have been rapid in recent years, making it difficult for reliable research to keep up with the pace (Tanner, 2006). From 10 programs in 1988 to the 230 accelerated BSN programs currently in operation (AACN, 2010), Wassem and Sheil's 1994 survey (as cited in Cangelosi & Whitt, 2005) identify accelerated program development issues that include "competition for clinical sites, heavy faculty workloads, program marketing, and poor screening of potential students" (p. 115). While accelerated nursing students are more mature learners who excel in class and are heavily praised by their employers (AACN, 2010), more research is needed on graduate outcomes and effectiveness of these programs beyond NCLEX-RN pass rates (Tanner, 2006). There is growing interest in the learning styles and preferences of second-degree students, along with recommendations for curriculum and program length (AACN, 2011; Cangelosi & Whitt, 2005; Tanner, 2006; Walker et al., 2007).

Issues and Challenges for Faculty

Faculty experience a variety of challenges with accelerated programming. Accelerated students typically demand more structure and guidance from faculty, often question relevance of and need for assignments, and are intolerant of busy work (Lindsey, 2009). For these reasons, experienced faculty may be better able to challenge students and meet the demands of teaching in this fast-paced program. Program administrators must address faculty workload and scheduling issues. For example, many accelerated programs run 12 months rather than the typical 9 months (Lindsey, 2009). Therefore, accelerated programming can present workload issues along with realistic budgetary concerns.

Teaching accelerated students can be challenging because of their maturity based on age, previous college experiences while earning a previous degree, and their ability to critically think and ask questions. Therefore, competent, resourceful faculty who are comfortable teaching diverse learners are integral in promoting these students' success (AACN, 2011).

Because accelerated programs are short in length, faculty challenges involve meeting both program and student demands (Suplee & Glasgow,

2008). Certainly teaching high volume, high quality, versus low volume, high quality makes teaching in accelerated programs demanding on faculty (Suplee & Glasgow, 2008).

Thus, teaching accelerated students requires faculty to enhance the learning environments and to develop teaching methodologies that fit with accelerated students' expectations and needs. In Rico, Beal, and Davies (2010), interviews of accelerated students reveal six themes that describe best faculty practices: "[faculty]. . . appreciate accelerated students as adult learners, communicate passion for the profession, challenge and motivate, practice while teaching and share their experiences, support accelerated students, and use varied teaching styles" (p. 150).

The Institute of Medicine's (2003) report, *Health Professions Education: A Bridge to Quality*, emphasizes EBP as an essential competency for all health care providers. Coupled with the Quality and Safety Education for Nurses (QSEN) initiative, nurse educators are mandated to prepare graduates who have the knowledge, skills, and attitudes to meet current clinical demands that reflect EBP (Cronenwett et al., 2007). Thus, the challenges to nurse educators are greater given the compressed curricular formats of accelerated, second-degree nursing programs.

Cangelosi (2007b) identified students' perceptions of the importance of clinical faculty during their accelerated program, noting that students ". . . admired and remembered the clinical instructors who sought out meaningful experiences for them as well. Capturing the pedagogical moment in routine and not-so-routine activities provided participants with the greatest links with their current nursing practice" (p. 403). This finding is significant since clinical faculty sometimes do not feel a part of the academic team or part of the clinical agencies where they teach (Brennan & Hutt, 2001).

Clinical instructors are often part-time faculty, which adds to the stress of the teaching role that may require orientation to multiple clinical agencies. In addition, the need to clarify course syllabi and multiple student requirements can add to the stress, making it increasingly difficult to effectively implement the clinical faculty role. Therefore, support from colleagues is essential to retain and promote quality clinical faculty and prevent them feeling at a lower status than tenured or tenure-track faculty (Brennan & Hutt, 2001; Kelly, 2006; Owen, 1993). Communication is the key element to facilitate positive faculty roles. Course orientations and course meetings to discuss concerns and issues allow clinical faculty input and promote ongoing, essential communication in accelerated program curricula.

Another challenge is the major shortage of nursing faculty nationwide. The AACN (2011) reports that nursing schools turned away

67,563 qualified applicants from both baccalaureate and graduate nursing programs in 2010 as a result of inadequate amounts of faculty, classroom space, clinical sites, preceptors, and budgetary constraints. Nearly two-thirds of schools pointed exclusively to faculty shortages as the main reason for not accepting every qualified applicant into their baccalaureate programs.

In 2008, the average age of nursing faculty in baccalaureate programs was 51.5 years, with typical retirement around age 62.5 (Allen, 2008). Today, with the average age of retirement for nurse faculty still at 62.5 years but the average age of doctorally prepared faculty at 53.5 years (AACN, 2011), a wave of faculty retirements is expected within the next 10 years.

According to AACN (2011) data, there is

"... a national nurse faculty vacancy rate of 6.9%. Most of the vacancies (90.6%) were faculty positions requiring or preferring a doctoral degree. The top reasons cited by schools having difficulty finding faculty were non-competitive salaries compared to positions in the practice arena (30.2%) and a limited pool of doctorally-prepared faculty (30.4%)" (Scope of the Nursing Faculty Shortage, para. 2.)

The major reasons that prevent schools of nursing from hiring more full-time faculty include insufficient funds, lack of college commitment for more full-time positions, competitive recruitment of faculty from other job markets, and unavailable qualified applicants in their geographic region (AACN, 2011). As the popularity of second-degree programs increase and faculty resources remain limited, schools of nursing will face difficult choices (Seldomridge & DiBartolo, 2005). Accelerated nursing programs require competent and willing faculty to teach second-degree students. Thus, maintaining faculty resources for traditional and accelerated programming presents a huge challenge for the future of nursing.

Issues and Challenges for Students

There are many issues and challenges for students entering an accelerated nursing program. The cost of an accelerated program can be unaffordable, and in a downward economy with limited funding resources, the inability to pay for school is a huge deterrent for many students wanting to enter an accelerated program (AACN, 2011). In 2005, Seldomridge and DiBartolo reported an average attrition rate of 10%, with an interesting 25% "no show" rate for accelerated students. Follow-up contact with the "no show" students revealed that their biggest reasons for not attending were financial considerations (Seldomridge & DiBartolo, 2005). In a subsequent study in 2007, the same authors found rising attrition rates to 23% of accelerated students, with one of the reasons for leaving including the need to work and make money (Seldomridge & DiBartolo, 2007).

Rouse and Rooda (2010) report that the majority of accelerated students work 20–40 hours per week to support themselves and their family. In an exit survey, one student commented, "... many people in the second-degree program also hold jobs. They are older, and many have children and need to work in order to scrape by" (Rouse & Rooda, 2010; p. 360). With continued economic uncertainty, there may be dramatic shifts in the demographics of students seeking admission to accelerated second-degree programs (Seldomridge & DiBartolo, 2005).

There are many other challenges for accelerated students in such fast-paced programs other than just costs. Other challenges include amount of commitment, time management, intense synthesis and application of knowledge, and the need to balance classroom, clinical, and life at home (Suplee & Glasgow, 2008). With accelerated programs ranging from 12 to 18 months versus the 3 years in traditional undergraduate nursing programs, the intensity is great and often contributes heavily to attrition (Cangelosi & Whitt, 2005). Nonacademic reasons for leaving the accelerated programs include the need for employment to help support the family, other family responsibilities, long commute times, and English as a second language (Rouse & Rooda, 2010).

Thus, the retention and attrition of accelerated second-degree students are vital issues that need to be addressed in research to better understand student populations and predict future enrollment management (Seldomridge & DiBartolo, 2005). According to the AACN (2011), some accelerated students struggle with the transition from being sophisticated, mature adults working in the real world to returning to life as a student in an undergraduate program. It is a tough transition that, according to Seldomridge and DiBartolo (2007), is in part due to the pace and intensity of the programs.

Specific ways to promote student retention include having an orientation program that provides realistic information about program demands and intensity, including schedules, allowing currently enrolled students or new graduates the opportunity to provide testimonials on how to prepare for program rigor, providing academic and psychological support services resources, creating focus group opportunities to foster communication, providing one-on-one faculty mentoring and advising, and providing avenues for financial assistance (Rouse & Rooda, 2010). Helping prospective students understand that these programs are accelerated, and not abbreviated, is crucial to helping decrease attrition rates (Meyer et al., 2006).

FUTURE DIRECTIONS

The success of accelerated nursing programs is dependent upon reliable research and qualified nursing faculty who understand the characteristics of diverse group of students that make up accelerated programs and teach well-designed courses (Suplee & Glasgow, 2008). With an increase in accelerated second-degree programs, it is crucial that new research continues to examine these programs. Specifically, answers to questions such as these are needed: Are accelerated programs improving the focus of nursing education? Are quicker programs still able to meet the learning needs of students? Should a different approach be used in the classroom or clinical setting? Are there long-term differences in traditional and accelerated graduates? How are quality indicators relative to patient outcomes affected by accelerated graduates? Are current second-degree accelerated nursing students significantly more diverse than their traditional counterparts? What are the factors that promote diversity in accelerated programs? How are accelerated students recruited and retained in accelerated programs? How do teachers and students experience accelerated nursing programs? What works and what does not work in current accelerated programs (Cangelosi & Whitt, 2005)? By failing to address these questions, the profession may be missing opportunities to make a career in nursing more accessible and move nurses into the workforce at a quicker pace (Ouellet & MacIntosh, 2007). The success of accelerated nursing programs is based upon well-designed and well-taught courses and programs (Suplee & Glasgow, 2008) that require continued research in order to move forward.

With regard to academics and the immense faculty shortage, there is a need for baccalaureate graduates who can quickly move into master's or doctoral degree programs and eventually into faculty roles (Lindsey, 2009). Since teaching accelerated students requires a high level of expertise from faculty, it is imperative that schools of nursing express the importance of quality teaching and clinical instruction. If clinical education is to remain strong, further research is needed that identifies strategies to recruit and retain nurse educators who can effectively blend the practice of teaching with the process of teaching (Cangelosi, 2007b).

Proven strategies to help make a smoother transition for new faculty should include mentoring programs and orientation sessions (Cangelosi, 2007a). It is also important to retain current faculty as a way to lessen the faculty shortage. Since many faculty are getting close to retirement, some feel overworked, and others leave education (AACN, 2011; Cangelosi, 2007b). Thus, an intervention such as providing monetary rewards for clinical expertise may be an effective way to retain faculty (Cangelosi, 2007b). Overall, it is essential that nurse educators adapt specific curricula and teaching strategies to meet the demands of second-degree nursing students, as they will comprise a good part of the clinical and academic leaders of tomorrow (Lindsey, 2009).

Second-degree nursing students are unique in many ways that include being motivated, academically gifted, and diverse (Seldomridge & DiBartolo, 2005). Over time, as the population changes, educational programs must be able to respond and adapt by considering alternative class and clinical schedules (Seldomridge & DiBartolo, 2005) and other types of programming. Therefore, knowing the characteristics of the accelerated student is very important for identifying the best recruitment strategies, along with dealing with retention and attrition issues. As the body of nursing knowledge grows around accelerated degree students, implementing specific retention interventions and evaluating their effectiveness will help aid in nursing student retention (Rouse & Rooda, 2010). Many other variables that affect a second-degree student, such as employment during school, family and home responsibilities, and postgraduation employer satisfaction (Seldomridge & DiBartolo, 2005) should be considered when designing programs and addressing retention interventions. Through evidence-based practice, accelerated nursing programs will be able to meet the special needs of second-degree students who "bring a wealth of knowledge, experience, and energy to the nursing workforce and are highly skilled clinicians" (AACN, 2010, Supporting Accelerated Nursing, para. 1).

REFERENCES

Allen, L. (2008). The nursing shortage continues as faculty shortage grows. *Nursing Economics, 26*(1), 35–40. Retrieved from EBSCO*host*.

American Association of Colleges of Nursing. (2010). *Accelerated programs: The fast-track to careers in nursing.* Retrieved from www.aacn.nche.edu/Publications/issues/Aug02.htm

American Association of Colleges of Nursing. (2011). Fact sheet: Nursing faculty shortage. Retrieved from http://www.aacn.nche.edu/Media/Factsheets/faculty shortage.htm

Brennan, A., & Hutt, R. (2001). The challenges and conflicts of facilitating learning in practice: The experiences of two clinical nurse educators. *Nurse Education in Practice, 1*, 181–188.

Bureau of Labor Statistics. (2010). Occupational employment projections to 2018. Retrieved from http://www.bls.gov/opub/mlr/2009/11/art5full.pdf

Bureau of Labor Statistics. (2011). Labor Force Statistics from the current population survey. Retrieved from http://www.bls.gov/cps/duration.htm

Cangelosi, P. (2007a). Accelerated second-degree baccalaureate nursing programs: What is the significance of clinical instructors? *Journal of Nursing Education, 46*(9), 400–405.

Cangelosi, P. (2007b). Voices of graduates from second-degree baccalaureate nursing programs. *Journal of Professional Nursing, 23*(2), 91–97. Retrieved from EBSCO*host.*

Cangelosi, P., & Whitt, K. (2005). Accelerated nursing programs: What do we know? *Nursing Education Perspectives, 26*(2), 113–116. Retrieved from CINAHL with Full Text database.

Cronenwett, L., Sherwood, G., Barnsteiner, J., Disch, J., Johnson, J., Mitchell, P. et al. (2007). Quality and safety education for nurses. *Nursing Outlook, 55,* 122–131.

Institute of Medicine. (2003). *Health professions education: A bridge to quality.* Washington, DC: National Academies Press.

Kelly, R. E. (2006). Engaging baccalaureate clinical faculty. *International Journal of Nursing Education Scholarship, 3*(1), 1–16.

Kruszewski, A., Brough, E., & Killeen, M. B. (2009). Collaborative strategies for teaching evidence-based practice in accelerated second-degree programs. *Journal of Nursing Education, 48*(6), 340–342.

Lindsey, P. (2009). Educational innovations. Starting an accelerated baccalaureate nursing program: Challenges and opportunities for creative educational innovations. *Journal of Nursing Education, 48*(5), 279–281. Retrieved from EBSCO*host.*

Meyer, G. A., Hoover, K. G., & Maposa, S. (2006). A profile of accelerated BSN graduates, 2004. *Journal of Nursing Education, 45*(8), 324–327.

Ouellet, L., & MacIntosh, J. (2007). The rise of accelerated baccalaureate programs. *Canadian Nurse, 103*(7), 28–31. Retrieved from EBSCO*host.*

Owen, S. (1993). Identifying a role for the nurse teacher in the clinical area. *Journal of Advanced Nursing, 13,* 816–825.

Penprase, B., & Koczara, S. (2009). Understanding the experiences of accelerated second-degree nursing students and graduates: A review of literature. *Journal of Continuing Education in Nursing, 40*(2), 74–78. Retrieved from CINAHL with Full Text database.

Rico, J. S., Beal, J., & Davies, T. (2010). Promising practices for faculty in accelerated nursing programs. *Journal of Nursing Education, 49*(3), 150–155.

Rouse, S., & Rooda, L. (2010). Factors for attrition in an accelerated baccalaureate nursing program. *Journal of Nursing Education, 49*(6), 359–362.

Saint Louis University Accelerated One-Year BSN: Introduction, n.d., para. 2. In Saint Louis University School of Nursing. Retrieved from http://www.slu.edu/x19741.xml

Seldomridge, L. A., & DiBartolo, M. C. (2005). A profile of accelerated second bachelor's degree nursing students. *Nurse Educator, 30*(2), 65–68.

Seldomridge, L. A., & DiBartolo, M. C. (2007). The changing face of accelerated second bachelor's degree students. *Nurse Educator, 32,* 240–245.

Suplee, D., & Glasgow, M. (2008). Curriculum innovation in an accelerated BSN program: The ACE model. *International Journal of Nursing Education Scholarship, 5*(1), 1–13.

Tanner, C. (2006). Changing times, evolving issues: The faculty shortage, accelerated programs, and simulation. *Journal of Nursing Education, 45*(3), 99–100. Retrieved from EBSCO*host*.

Walker, J., Martin, T., Haynie, L., Norwood, A., White, J., & Grant, L. (2007). Preferences for teaching methods in a baccalaureate nursing program: How second-degree and traditional students differ. *Nursing Education Perspectives, 28*(5), 246–250. Retrieved from CINAHL with Full Text database.

Chapter

2

Curriculum Innovation

Mahmoud Kaddoura, Collette Williams, and Terri Jabaley

INTRODUCTION

*C*urriculum development in nursing education is an innovative process that aims at generating an integrated, meaningful nursing curriculum. The goal of curriculum innovation is to create learning opportunities, which will build students' professional knowledge and skills so that graduate nurses will practice nursing competently in an ever-changing health care environment. In this way, curriculum innovation contributes to the health and quality of life of the clients served by nursing students and the patients nursing graduates serve (Iwasiw, Goldenberg, & Andrusyszyn, 2009). The need for innovation in nursing education through the nursing curriculum development and redesigning process is crucial to cope with the rapidly changing health care delivery system. It is widely noted in the literature that because of the complexity of today's health care system and health care delivery, transformation of nursing education is a necessity (American Association of Colleges of Nursing, 2008; Bellack, 2008; Coonan, 2008).

For years, nursing has debated about curriculum reform and innovation. Currently, there is both a shortage of nurses and a lack of adequate preparation of nurses in terms of critical thinking, problem solving, and clinical decision-making skills to work in today's health care system (American Association of Colleges of Nursing, 2008). Today's nursing education prepares students at multiple levels for practice entry through diploma, associate, and baccalaureate degrees. Traditional curricular approaches predominate, using a segmented, course-by-course approach to teaching, often without thoughtful and planned integration of pertinent concepts across courses and throughout the curriculum. Some of these pervasive and essential concepts include ethical considerations, genetics and genomics, informatics, and cultural diversity. The future of nursing education needs to focus on changing demographics of health care, preparing students to meet the highly technological, diverse, ever-changing, and evidence-based structure of the real world of health care today. There is growing awareness that knowledge quickly evolves in nursing, and thus the nursing curriculum needs to be open and flexible, utilizing interdisciplinary studies and integrating essential concepts across the curriculum (NLN, 2005).

Various factors constitute the compelling forces behind curriculum innovation in nursing education. In nursing education, moving away from teacher-centered to student-centered classrooms has been a crucial necessity in developing the type of health professional that is needed today (Glennon, 2006). Nurse educators are called upon to take a critical perspective toward the way curriculum is designed and operationalized, determining its shortcomings and areas of needed improvement to meet the needs of rapidly changing health care environments (NLN, 2005). In this chapter, the authors present a review of literature related to curriculum innovation in accelerated nursing education and discuss challenges and strategies to design and implement innovative curriculum in an accelerated program. Future direction of curriculum innovation in accelerated nursing education is suggested.

REVIEW OF THE LITERATURE

Nursing education is in the process of transformation influenced by a number of factors, including the widespread use of new technologies, the serious shortage of nurse faculty, and the realization that today's nursing students are a diverse group with multiple learning styles. Faculty are challenged to capture the attention of the learner, to focus on what the learner knows, and to engage students in their own individual learning experiences. It is important to note that faculty and students may have different views of what constitutes innovative teaching. For the National League for Nursing (NLN) Task Group on Innovation in Nursing Education, innovation is the use of knowledge to create ways and services that are perceived as new to transform systems (National League for

Nursing, 2005). It requires challenging long-held assumptions and values. The outcome of innovation in nursing education is excellence in nursing practice and the development of a culture that supports risk-taking, creativity, and excellence (Pardue et al., 2005).

Traditional methods of nursing education need to give way to more innovative approaches to prepare graduate nurses with competent experiences for their future nursing practice. The National Council of State Boards of Nursing (2009) defines innovation as a dynamic, systematic process that envisions new approaches to nursing education. The literature reported curricular innovations that include the use of dedicated education units for clinical education (Moscato, Miller, Logsdon, Weinberg, & Chorpenning, 2007), educational approaches such as narrative pedagogy and deliberate discussion (Goodin & Stein, 2008), and high-fidelity simulation as an adjunct to or replacement for clinical experiences (Reese, Jeffries, & Engun, 2010). Other innovations in nursing education include partnering with clinical agencies or with other educational institutions to share resources for the delivery of nursing education.

Nursing, along with the environments in which nurses' work, has been changing rapidly due to the fast-paced advancement in health care technology, the use and complexity of information and communications. These changes in nursing practice necessitate changes in nursing education. Among the various strategies proposed, one innovative approach to nursing education is the accelerated degree program for nonnursing graduates. Offered at the baccalaureate degree level, these programs build on previous learning experiences and provide a way for individuals with undergraduate degrees in other disciplines to transition into nursing, according to the American Association of Colleges of Nursing (2010). Accelerated nursing programs are the fastest growing to meet the looming nursing workforce crisis needs. When enrolling in accelerated nursing programs, hard work and focus is definitely needed. Coursework can be very demanding, since it is a compressed curriculum of what traditional students take in a four- or five-year course of study. Even though the time frame is less, the content and quality of classroom teaching, laboratory experiences, and actual exposure in hospitals and other health care facilities are relatively the same. The opportunities for graduates of accelerated nursing programs, after successful completion of the licensing examination, are equal to those of traditional graduates. Accelerated second-degree baccalaureate programs offer the quickest route to licensure as a registered nurse (RN) for those who have already completed a non-nursing bachelor's or graduate degree. Accelerate baccalaureate programs in nursing take between 11 and 18 months to complete, including prerequisites (Raines, 2010).

The first accelerated second-degree baccalaureate nursing program was offered in 1971 at St. Louis University. Students in this program could complete a BSN degree in one year (Domrose, 2001). Prestigious institutions such as Johns Hopkins University have offered accelerated programs within schools of nursing that can be completed in 13 months (Shiber, 2003). The abundance of these programs during the past two decades has been exceptional. Components of successful second-degree accelerated programs include utilizing the experiences of students with previous degrees and offering flexible clinical courses more than once each calendar year. Shiber (2003) described the accelerated student as a "capable person who knows why learning is required [and] will find a way to acquire that learning independently in a personally meaningful way" (p. 136). In 2009, there were 230 accelerated baccalaureate programs available at nursing schools nationwide. More new accelerated baccalaureate programs are in the planning stages. The American Association of Colleges of Nursing (AACN) 2009 survey found that 11,930 students were enrolled in accelerated baccalaureate programs, up from 11,018, 9,938, 8,493, 7,829, and 6,090 students in 2008, 2007, 2006, 2005, and 2004, respectively. The number of program graduates has also increased with 7,444 graduates in 2009 as compared to 6,870, 5,881, 5,232, 3,769, and 2,422 graduates in 2008, 2007, 2006, 2005, and 2004, respectively (AACN 2010).

The proliferation of accelerated nursing programs has further prompted the need for nursing education reform. Such reform calls for new educational pedagogies that move away from the traditional approach, providing new educational pedagogies that result in positive outcomes and meet the needs of learners, and health care providers as employers of future nurses (American Association of Colleges of Nursing, 2010; Institute of Medicine, 2010).

CHALLENGES

Nursing curricula have been challenged to meet the varied learning needs of students of the new century, in an evolving, complex society. With the Bureau of Labor Statistics prediction that 1 million new registered nurses will be needed by 2012, the pressure is on to find rapid and effective ways to educate large numbers of RNs (American Association of Colleges of Nursing, 2010). Some challenges of note in accelerated programs include lack of financial aid for accelerated students and the potential for animosity between traditional and accelerated students. Despite these challenges, successful accelerated programs were viewed as a model for curriculum innovation. Reasons for the rapid growth of these programs are numerous but primarily include the need for more nurses in response to the current and projected nursing shortage and the necessity of more baccalaureate-prepared nurses (Cangelosi & Whitt, 2005). Nursing programs have increased recruitment strategies to attract more students to the profession, with accelerated second-degree programs being one such strategy (Shiber, 2003). The question remains, how do we, in a brief period of time, educate nurses who have the ability to deliver quality patient care in a dynamic and complex environment? The following are identified challenges to innovative nursing curricula.

Regulatory Challenges to Innovative Nursing Curricula

The changing panorama of health care in America requires that nursing students and future nurses be skilled in responding to varying patient expectations and values; provide ongoing patient management; deliver and coordinate care across teams, settings, and time frames; and support patients' endeavors to change behavior and lifestyle in today's academic and clinical settings (Institute of Medicine, 2010). Nursing education needs to innovate at the micro- and macrosystem levels for the 21st century. In order to truly transform care, practice and education will need to partner on curriculum development and the professional socialization of the new nurse. Background Innovation in academic settings, specifically colleges of nursing, is often hindered by the pressure to meet educational and regulatory requirements established by national organizations, accrediting agencies, and the state boards of nursing that govern and set standards for nursing practice at the baccalaureate levels (Melnyk & Davidson, 2009). These regulations should not be barriers to innovation. Time-honored traditions in nursing education, such as the current undergraduate clinical instruction model, a disease and illness-oriented curriculum, and the need for extensive clinical practice before matriculating in graduate programs, should be reexamined.

Although innovation in nursing education is a must to meet the future needs of nurses and the demands of the ever-changing health care environment, when planning an innovative curriculum, faculty should be aware of potential challenges that may hinder the implementation of curricular innovations. There may be regulatory challenges to innovation in nursing education. Potential regulatory challenges may include a specific number of clinical or didactic hours in the nursing curriculum. Other challenges may encompass faculty–student ratios, full-time and part-time ratios of faculty in a nursing program, and simulation limitations (NCSBN, 2009).

Advanced knowledge of potential challenges may help faculty in negotiating with stakeholders to overcome these challenges and create innovative curricula that forward thinking on educating nurses for the future. Thinking about the consequences of and compliance with the individual state nurse practice act and state nursing regulations before planning or redesigning innovative curricular changes is very important (Hargreaves, 2008).

Managing Essential Content in Nursing Curricula

There are many challenges for participants in accelerated programs, including the amount of work, time management, synthesis and application of knowledge, building and retaining knowledge, and balancing classroom, clinical, and home life. An important challenge for teaching in accelerated second-degree programs is how to manage essential content within a compressed curriculum format.

Today's nursing curriculum is dense, and integrating new content is a challenge. Since it is integral and critical to all areas of nursing practice to incorporate various principles such as geriatric patient care, clinical simulation, genetic and genomic information, and so on, nursing curricula must prepare graduates with this information (Williams, 2002).

Practice and curriculum change require the commitment of nursing leaders and academic faculty to develop a long-term plan to incorporate genetic and genomic information in order to improve public health. Faculty and practicing nurses must be supported by their institutions to attend continuing education or academic courses to update their genetic and genomic knowledge. Collaboration with other disciplines is necessary to provide a strong foundation of knowledge of basic human genetics and current applications to practice. Essential content in nursing curricula should be consistent with national priorities of health care reform. An innovative nursing curriculum should include theoretical and practical content to ensure skills appropriate for the application of the content. Values-based leadership should also be integrated into the curriculum to ensure that nursing graduates are fully prepared to be safe and competent nurses and to lead health care in the 21st century. Additionally, interdisciplinary educational learning experiences should be emphasized to prepare nurses who have the potential to be future health leaders. Innovative curricular faculty should incorporate diverse disciplines in their content and all learning experiences to emphasize the value of interdisciplinary practice in the nursing curriculum (American Nurses Association, 2004).

The innovative nursing curriculum requires content selection criteria to reflect the relationship of course content to program outcomes, one of which is caring. Nursing educators and practicing nurses include items within the areas of commonly encountered health problems, ethical issues, chronic illness, long-term care of older adults, and nursing process. Therefore, gerontological nursing content is crucial to innovative nursing curricula that faculty should integrate all through the curriculum (American Association of Colleges of Nursing, 2008).

Diversity in Student Population

Today's student population is very different from that in the past. The millennium has become the symbol for the extraordinary challenges and opportunities available to the nursing profession and to those academic institutions responsible for preparing the next generation of nurses. Transformations taking place in nursing and nursing education have been driven by major socioeconomic factors, as well as by developments in health care delivery and professional issues unique to nursing. These changes have shaped the move toward increased diversity of both patients and student population in our world today, and provided new and different opportunities and challenges from those of the past. Changing demographics and increasing diversity have an important impact on nursing education (Bradshaw & Lowenstein, 2010).

Population shifts in the United States have affected health care priorities as well as the practice of nursing. Due to advances in public health and clinical care, the average lifespan is increasing rapidly. By 2020, more than 20% of the population will be 65 and older, with those over 85 constituting the fastest-growing age group. Greater life expectancy of individuals with chronic and acute conditions will challenge the health care system's ability to provide efficient and effective continuing care. Significant increases in the diversity of the population affect the nature and the prevalence of illness and disease, requiring changes in practice that reflect and respect diverse values and beliefs. Nursing education, practice, and research must embrace and respond to these changing demographics, and nurses must focus on spiritual health, as well as the physical and psychosocial health of the population. The nursing classroom is more diverse than ever before. Yet, diversity no longer means ethnic background alone. The age range may be wide and the gender ratios may have changed, although nursing still has a minority of male students (Bradshaw & Lowenstein, 2010).

Student demographics are also changing. Ethnic and racial diversity of nursing schools has increased dramatically, creating a rich cultural environment for learning. Students are entering schools of nursing at an older age and are bringing varying college and work experiences, as well as more sophisticated expectations for their education. They are typically employed in full-time careers, and many are raising families, which places constraints on their educational experiences and necessitates greater flexibility in scheduling. Schools of nursing must be prepared to confront the challenges associated with today's more mature student body, educational methods and policies, curriculum and case materials, clinical practice settings, and research priorities need to value and reflect the diversity of the student body, as well as the population in general. Research reveals that second-degree students bring with them a high level of maturity and previous life experiences that involve critical thinking. Such experience is thought to increase their ability to make competent professional decisions (Cangelosi, 2007). Current research shows that compared to students in traditional nursing programs, accelerated students tend to be older, married, highly motivated, and more often male (American Association of Colleges of Nursing 2008). After second-degree students graduate, employers report high levels of satisfaction with their performance, as they tend to be strong problem solvers, have a greater maturity with a variety of life experiences, and become lifelong learners (Beal, 2007).

Classroom in Innovative Curricula

The use of the term "innovation" in discussions related to nursing curriculum and classroom has become widespread. There are various reasons why classroom activities need to be innovative. It is assumed that through curriculum changes, students could enjoy learning and improve their academic achievement. Innovative classroom strategies should focus on improving students' motivation and engagement and develop their independence and working in teams. They should include skills that are necessary for students' learning through application of the content covered in their curriculum in clinical settings. Such application of knowledge is crucial for students' future career as well as for their professional and personal development.

The types of teaching methods used by faculty in the classroom setting depend on many variables, including familiarity of the strategy. Traditional lecture, which follows the pedagogical model of teacher-centered education, was found in the review of literature to be the most utilized teaching method by faculty in classrooms today. Many faculty use lecture as a primary teaching method in part because they are most familiar with it. According to Hartman, Dziuban, and Brophy-Ellison (2007), approximately 80% of college instruction occurs utilizing lecture.

In their study, Johnson and Mighten (2005) attempted to identify the most effective teaching methods for nursing students by comparing two teaching strategies: lecture only versus lecture notes combined with structured group discussion. The study included 169 nursing students taking a medical–surgical nursing course in an urban college of nursing. All students were divided into two groups; a control group ($n = 88$) and an experimental group ($n = 81$). The control group received lecture as the only teaching method for the entire course, while the experimental group received lecture notes one week in advance and then participated in group discussions over the material during class (Johnson & Mighten, 2005). Overall, those in the experimental group who participated in group discussions during class had significantly higher examination scores with fewer course failures than those in the control group who were exposed to lecture only (Johnson & Mighten, 2005). The findings of this study support the use of a variety of teaching methods. According to Johnson and Mighten (2005) "traditional lecture is not the most effective teaching method" and a combination of teaching strategies is necessary to ensure success in nursing education (p. 321).

Motivation of Nursing Students

As schools of nursing look to the future of the accelerated education of students, they must also look to motivating these students and meeting their learning needs. The accelerated nursing curricula need to move from a pedagogical approach to an andragogical approach. Pedagogy is based on teacher-centered and teacher-directed learning in which teachers select the applicable topics and determine the structure of the teaching-learning process. The teacher's role in this approach is to impart knowledge and the students' role is like a vessel; to passively receive the imparted knowledge. This model of teaching often embraces the lecture-based model (Connor, 2003). Innovation in nursing curricula requires empowering and nurturing students in order to promote adult learning. Learning occurs most effectively when competent nursing educators assume the role of facilitators during the teaching–learning process and partner with students and other health care professionals. These adult learners may need some direction to be responsible for their own learning as they move from pedagogy to andragogy. Nursing educators who demonstrate genuineness, compassion, empathy, and respect for their students best model professionalism and inspire the learner. Diversity of the student population adds to the richness of the learning environment with all its experiences, including student motivation. Students need to be motivated by becoming active learners who are engaged in their own lifelong learning. Moreover, the role of the faculty needs to include motivating students, challenging them, and providing opportunities for them to learn. Faculty need to move away from content-driven curricula to what students need in order to function in today's health care settings. Process-driven curriculum focuses on learning strategies and thinking processes rather than on content. The challenges of nurse educators lie in changing their instructional method from a teacher-centered, content-driven approach to this learner-centered, process-driven approach. Content-driven curricula (which describe many nursing curricula) emphasize "covering content" more than student learning, students' excitement about learning, processes, values development, and so on. The curricula need to provide experiential learning opportunities and assessments of learning outcomes in order to ensure that the outcomes are positive (Candela, Dalley, & Benzel-Lindley, 2006).

Students must be able to apply the knowledge being learned in the classroom for professional practice in their clinical practicum. This can be challenging as the nursing student body nowadays is different. The majority of accelerated students pose challenges for students, faculty, and schools of nursing. These older students tend to be more self-directed in their learning. The attempt to assimilate these students with traditional students in the same classroom adds an additional challenge for faculty. Challenges facing schools of nursing are the varied demographic mix, meeting the needs of different types of learners in one classroom, increased pool of qualified applicants, and the usual challenge of finding clinical placements. The complexity and challenge of teaching the large amount of content to a diverse student body while meeting the needs of students with different learning styles can be daunting. Nursing curricula need to be innovative in order to meet students' various learning needs (Bradshaw & Lowenstein, 2010).

One major detriment to student engagement involves the concept of academic motivation. Ironside and Valiga (2006) claimed the topic of student laziness, noncommittal attitudes, and general lack of respect predominate informal conversations among nurse faculty. Several factors have been shown to foster student motivation. Student observation of positive consequences as a result of peers' efforts was believed to encourage motivation, at least in the short-term (Schunk, 2004). Along with rewarding outcomes, personal belief in one's abilities was shown to contribute to more sustained levels of motivation (Schunk, 2004). In addition

TABLE 2.1 Summary of Challenges, Strategies, and Future Directions for Curricular Innovation

CHALLENGES	STRATEGIES	FUTURE DIRECTIONS
Regulatory challenges to innovative nursing curricula	Accelerated nursing program as an innovative curricular approach	Use of clinical partnerships
Managing essential content in nursing curricula	The Accelerated Career Entry (ACE) Model	Integrated Curriculum Model
Diversity in student population	EBP Model	Coach, Preceptor, Mentor Team (CPMT) Model
Classroom in innovative curricula	Use of technology in the classroom	Use of student-centered active teaching strategies to meet learning needs
Motivation of nursing students	Experiential learning	

to self-efficacy, the expectation for success and control orientation, or the perceived level of control learners have over their learning environments were also factors in motivation (Lynch, 2006). The generation of current traditional college students, meaning those born from the early 1980s on, are products of the times. They reflect patterns of increased consumption, consistent and oftentimes intensive parental attention compared to previous generations, and allegiance to web-surfing, online relationships, and harboring group mentality (Crone & MacKay, 2007). One recent survey found that the general perception among nursing faculty was that "students in their program 'are excited about learning and exhibit a spirit of inquiry and a sense of wonderment'" (Ironside & Valiga, 2006, p. 168). Nursing education has recognized that student needs continue to evolve. Faculty are challenged to find ways to more actively engage students in their education. Table 2.1 provides a summary of the curricular innovation challenges of accelerated nursing programs.

STRATEGIES

Typically, accelerated baccalaureate nursing programs shorten the amount of time to educate entry-level nurses. This is partially accomplished by changing the educational paradigm from traditional pedagogy to a student-centered learning approach. Pardue et al. (2005) noted that although there have been innovations in nursing education, much of what has been described is a rearrangement of content from one course or semester to another. Few designs for paradigm-shifting changes in nursing curriculum are present in the literature. It appears that "nurse educators continue to attempt to teach in ways that they were taught" (Pardue et al., 2005, p. 55).

Accelerated Nursing Curriculum as an Innovative Curricular Approach

One innovative approach to nursing education that is gaining momentum nationwide is the accelerated baccalaureate degree program for non-nursing graduates (Cangelosi & Whitt, 2005). According to the AACN (2008), accelerated programs build on previous learning experiences and transition individuals with undergraduate degrees in other disciplines into nursing. Nursing curricula in accelerated programs prepare students for essential roles and responsibilities to practice safe and quality nursing care.

The accelerated curriculum design requires a full-time commitment as it compresses 4 years of full-time study into an average of about 15 months (the most common program lengths in general include the minimum of 11 months and the maximum of 18 months) of a program of study. Most of the accelerated nursing programs in the United States are offered to the second-degree students. The generic accelerated BSN program was offered at the Massachusetts College of Pharmacy and Health Sciences (MCPHS) in Boston, Massachusetts in 2005. This program is designed in a 32-month year-round format. Each of the first 2 years of the curriculum consists of 15-week fall and spring semesters and a 10- or 12-week summer session. The third year consists of 15-week fall and spring semesters and concludes in May. The curriculum requires 125 semester hours of credit for completion, which includes the general education core curriculum requirements common to all MCPHS undergraduate and first professional degree programs, additional professional support courses in the natural and social sciences, and courses in the nursing major. On completion of the program, students are eligible to sit for the National Council of State Boards of Nursing Licensure Examination for Registered Nurses (NCLEX-RN).

In addition to these face-to-face types of accelerated programs, there are at least 100 online institutions that offer accelerated BSN programs. Moreover, there are some hybrid accelerated BSN programs in which part of the courses are offered online and a significant part is offered in face-to-face classes. The major intent of accelerated nursing programs is to attract students with a baccalaureate or higher degree in fields other than nursing and nontraditional, mature individuals seeking a second career.

The Accelerated Career Entry (ACE) Model

An additional innovative curriculum includes the Accelerated Career Entry (ACE) Program, which was originally created by Drexel University to address the challenges associated with accelerated nursing programs and to reduce the attrition rate. The ACE Program was initially formed by two faculty members in 2000 to contribute to alleviating the nursing shortage and provide adult learners with avenues to obtain a baccalaureate nursing degree other than the traditional 4-year option (Suplee & Glasgow, 2008).

The ACE Program was designed to educate nurses for providing care for individuals in health, illness, and through some of life's most difficult transitions. This design was based on the original undergraduate nursing program with 21–23 credits per quarter. The program was adjusted to the preexisting academic calendar of 11 months (Suplee & Glasgow, 2008). Courses not traditionally found in undergraduate nursing curricula that were included in the ACE Model were Nursing Informatics, Genetics in Nursing and Health, and Contemporary Gerontological Nursing. A capstone course, Senior Seminar, was designed for the final quarter, and incorporated a review for the Registered Nurse licensure exam (NCLEX-RN exam), a Standardized Patient Experience, and a demonstration of core clinical competencies (Suplee & Glasgow, 2008).

Evidence-Based Practice (EBP) Model

The literature clearly calls for more innovation in nursing education and the commitment of nursing faculty to implement innovative, evidence-based approaches to teaching and learning (Bellack, 2008; Coonan, 2008; Dreher, 2008; Ironside & Valiga, 2007; Tanner, 2008). EBP in nursing is the means by which a patient receives nursing care; *education* reflects the acquisition of the nursing knowledge and skills necessary to become a proficient clinician and to maintain competency; and *research* provides new knowledge to the profession and enables the development of practices based on scientific evidence. The goal of EBP in nursing is to promote improved interventions, care, and patient outcomes. Current curricular innovation has focused on EBP in nursing, which integrates the use of current best evidence with nurses' clinical expertise and patient preferences in the clinical setting to deliver optimal care (Cronenwett et al., 2007). Nursing students at all levels need to bring themselves into nursing in the 21st century by applying EBP in real-world scenarios. The mandate for nurse educators is to prepare graduates with the knowledge, skills, and attitudes to meet the requirements for current clinical practice. The Quality and Safety Education for Nurses (QSEN) project (Cronenwett et al., 2007) listed EBP as one of the six competencies for quality and safety education in nursing programs.

According to Ironside and Valiga (2007), the EBP curriculum provides learning experiences that prepare graduates to assume roles that are essential to quality nursing practice, including but not limited to roles of care provider, patient advocate, teacher, communicator, change agent, care coordinator, user of information technology, collaborator, and decision maker. Faculty decide what type of evidence should be introduced at what level. For instance, in introductory nursing courses, the EBP concept is defined and students are asked to do a literature search on basic skills such as hand washing or universal precautions. Later in the curriculum, students may be asked to review literature based on sample sizes or types of studies to gain insight into when practice should be changed based on the evidence (Suplee & Glasgow, 2008).

Use of Technology in the Classroom

Since the 1970s, there has been rapid growth and development in instructional technology use guided by research on teaching, learning, and cognitive science in general (Leinonen & Järvelä, 2006). The emerging technology represents a shift from the predominantly behaviorist pedagogy (teacher-centered) to a more constructivist approach (student-centered). The constructivist approach focuses on facilitating deep, integrated, and conceptual learning, rather than focusing on discrete and compartmentalized knowledge and skills (Ferguson & Day, 2005). Constructivist pedagogy emphasizes active learning strategies by engaging the student in authentic activities that model real-world scenarios and practitioner behavior (Ferguson & Day, 2005). In the context of nursing, such competencies are critical for the provision of optimal patient care. Among the instructional technology tools used in nursing education, much attention is given to simulation learning technology as supportive of this paradigm shift in education (Spunt, Dawn, & Adams, 2004).

According to Kaddoura (2010), simulation incorporates scenarios and case studies developed to replicate real-life clinical situations, in which learners are asked to solve clinical problems and make critical decisions based on provided information. It is an instructional tool intended to engender certain skills and knowledge sets so that the nurse can be better prepared to provide optimal patient care.

The rapid growth in information technology has a radical impact on health care delivery and nurse education. Kaddoura (2010) conducted a study to explore the perceptions of new graduate nurses on how clinical simulation developed their critical thinking, learning, and confidence throughout their clinical training. The nurses stated that simulation enhanced their critical thinking and skill acquisition in a safe and user-friendly environment, and prepared them well to care confidently for critically ill patients. Simulation also helped them learn to make sound clinical decisions to improve patient outcomes. The findings of this study provide evidence to support the use of simulation as a teaching strategy to promote critical thinking, learning, and confidence (Kaddoura, 2010).

Technology influences every educational discipline, including nursing. To cope with the fast-paced advancement in technology, classrooms are equipped with technology and faculty development activities that include training on educational technology applications. Integration of technology in classroom, computer literacy by nursing faculty and students, and information technology are crucial in nursing curricula and professional practice (American Association of Colleges of Nursing, 2010). The use of technology could enhance the profession's ability to educate nurses for practice, prepare future nurse educators, and advance nursing science in an era when the number of professional nurses, qualified nurse faculty, and nurse researchers is well below national needs (American Association of Colleges of Nursing, 2010).

Today's nurses utilize high-tech equipment at the bedside and to address the need for understanding and utilizing health informatics to assist in determining the best practices in health care delivery. In order to demonstrate competent care, nurses today need to incorporate the use of technology in the acute care, long-term care, and community settings. Health care technology allows for nurses to employ current data at the point of care in making nursing decisions with regard to patient care. The use of technology allows for the management of data and information to assist with clinical decision making. Patient safety and quality patient care have always been the cornerstone of nursing practice. The use of technology allows for the analysis of date, which allows for better decision making, quality improvement strategies, and support of evidence-based care (Institute of Medicine, 2010).

Nursing faculty strive to use best practices in their teaching in the classroom, the laboratory, and clinical settings. One way to achieve this is by integrating various teaching methodologies. In addition to the traditional PowerPoint presentation as the most commonly chosen method for teaching, technological devices used in accelerated classrooms may include the use of clickers and personal digital assistants (PDAs) for classroom and clinical settings. Students receive a clicker and a PDA during orientation and learn to use them, specifically to download provided texts; use and access Blackboard; access data through electronic texts; perform library searches; and access information at the point of care—the bedside. "Providing students with the opportunity to practice accessing and utilizing relevant information in clinical settings can, in turn, support the development of clinical competency and clinical decision making skills" (Glasgow & Cornelius, 2005, p. 176).

Experiential Learning

Experiential learning is built into the curriculum in an accelerated BSN program. Experiential learning involves incorporating the use of simulation in the Health Assessment and Nursing Skills course, which have laboratory components to enhance student learning. The standardized patient lab experience has been a useful means to assess outcomes and to provide both formative and summative evaluations for students in the lab. Students are provided a short patient history and then enter an exam room. Depending on the case scenario, students obtain a history, perform a physical assessment, and provide patient education, with a trained actor as the patient. Students are videotaped and their performance is evaluated by the actors, faculty members, and students themselves. Student–patient interactions and communication skills are highlighted throughout the experience (Suplee & Glasgow, 2008).

There is usually a pass/fail grade for lab courses, and students are provided with remediation and another opportunity to complete this experience at a later date if they are unsuccessful; however, most students are successful the first time. Faculty appreciate the experience since it gives an insight into the communication and skill performance abilities of students. Students generally do not rate these experiences highly because it is stress producing; yet, they find it useful. Although this type of evaluation is more costly, the ultimate benefits outweigh the costs, as traditional methods of evaluation may not truly represent the means for assessing clinical competency (Ebbertt & Connors, 2004). Table 2.1 provides a summary of the curricular innovation strategies used in accelerated nursing programs.

FUTURE DIRECTIONS

The literature related to accelerated, or second-degree, nursing programs and students reveals that the demand for these programs has increased dramatically in the past several years. Nursing knowledge is expanding considerably, and health care practice is changing rapidly. New challenges in practice include an aging population, a shift from acute to chronic diseases in patients and therefore in nursing treatment models, increasing attention to patient safety and quality of care, and recurrent calls to decrease health care costs. The locations of health care delivery are moving from hospital to community settings, resulting in increased inpatient acuity and diminished availability of traditional clinical teaching sites. Student demographics have also shifted, and new technology offers alternative delivery systems. The curricular innovation has focused on the addition or rearrangement of content within the curriculum, rather than on significant, paradigm shift-type changes (National League for Nursing, 2005).

The nursing shortage has been a vital challenge for hospitals and academic institutions offering nursing programs. These challenges have stimulated colleges and universities to develop and promote accelerated programs in an effort to recruit nontraditional students into nursing. In the interim, nursing curricula are already overloaded, and it is difficult to imagine adding yet more content. Both classroom and clinical teaching systems pose challenges in the current environment. A new system for the integration of these two domains is needed, along with greater support for the transition from education to practice. Making these issues even more challenging are the concurrent faculty shortages and the current economic crisis. Nonetheless, educators and clinicians are in agreement about the need for curricular innovation, if not about the details of needed change. All levels of nursing education, undergraduate and graduate, are obligated to challenge their long-held traditions and design evidence-based curricula that are flexible, responsive to students' needs, collaborative, and integrate current technology. Faculty, students, consumers, and nursing service personnel must work in partnership to design innovative educational systems that meet the needs of the health care delivery system now and in the future (National League for Nursing, 2005). Based on the challenges and strategies identified, many ideas emerge that are worthy of more detailed scrutiny in innovative nursing curricula.

Use of Clinical Partnerships

Innovative curricula in nursing colleges and universities across the country require creative solutions to increase the number of registered nurses in response to the growing shortage. Budgetary constraints, a limited pool of nursing faculty, insufficient clinical sites, and a lack of scholarship monies are all barriers to expanding student capacity and meeting the projected demand for nursing care. To overcome these challenges, nursing institutions should collaborate with clinical partners in an effort to build student capacity and satisfy mutual needs. These partnerships take many forms and serve various functions. Some schools use expert practitioners to augment the nursing faculty supply. Others involve collaborative arrangements among nursing education programs to increase student enrollments. Some service partners share physical resources and infrastructure with schools as a means of overcoming limitations in clinical, classroom, and research space. Still others form partnerships to provide tuition forgiveness to students in exchange for work commitments.

The role of the clinical instructor in innovative nursing curricula has changed to bridge theory into practice. Nursing faculty take a great responsibility in the professional development of nursing students. Since the shift of nursing to a more academic setting, nursing faculty have had to develop a collaborative practice with clinical faculty in providing the application of nursing theory taught in the classroom to clinical practice. The data currently show that there is a national faculty vacancy rate of 6.9% (American Association of Colleges of Nursing, 2010). Many schools of nursing have adapted a clinical partnership model that allows for bringing theory taught in the classroom to the clinical site by employing nurse educators to oversee the student clinical experience. These clinical faculty are not only teaching the students but are also acting as mentors, providing professional socialization and aids in the professional development of students.

Integrated Curriculum Model

Despite the plethora of literature on accelerated programs, there is a lack of consensus on what constitutes an accelerated nursing program. If, as the AACN report (2008) suggests, these programs continue to increase at a greater rate than traditional nursing programs, it is important that nurse educators identify the best methods for educating and advising these students (Schreier, Peery, & McLean, 2009).

Integrated nursing curricula should have a philosophy that, by integrating many different disciplines into nursing curriculum and by working with professionals with many different skills, nurses can provide better care to patients after being licensed. Nursing colleges and universities that adopt integrated nursing curricula are expected to provide a more generalized approach to nursing to cover many areas, and they emphasize a team-nursing approach. Many traditional programs attempt to integrate various concepts such as nutrition or geriatrics in their course work. This has led to limited success, as the concepts are often integrated inconsistently.

As an alternative, some colleges use curriculum models defining nursing as the holistic care of individuals, families, and communities. Courses are developed that incorporated concepts across the lifespan rather than traditional maternal–child, mental health, and adult medical–surgical courses. Curriculum strands may include oxygenation, circulation, metabolism, immunity, cognition and perception, mobility, elimination, and sexuality and reproduction (Schreier et al., 2009). Threads may include health appraisal, challenges to health care, disease, nutrition, ethical and legal issues, leadership and management, diversity, environment, communication, roles, and psychosocial issues. Classroom concepts are coordinated with clinical and laboratory experiences to enhance the integration of knowledge. Students' beginning didactic and clinical experiences may involve assessments of surrounding communities. Subsequent didactic and clinical experiences include family assessment with dyads of students assigned to families (Schreier et al., 2009). After this initial phase, didactic and laboratory experiences focus on nursing care of the individual. Clinical skills are taught in the first semester and the first week of the second semester. As the concept threads begin with oxygenation, the laboratory experiences begin with associated skills such as assessment of the respiratory system and oxygen therapy. In the second semester, students are fully prepared to practice skills in the clinical setting (Schreier et al., 2009).

Coach, Preceptor, Mentor Team (CPMT) Model

The clinical experience provides opportunities to apply nursing knowledge and address clinical competencies. In the CPMT model, the team is composed of the faculty member, the student, and the preceptor. Preceptors attend a specialized training workshop presented by faculty. Each faculty member is assigned to 10 students, and each student is assigned to a preceptor on a selected hospital unit. Students work one-on-one with preceptors to deliver patient care. Faculty visit students regularly and are always available by pager to students and preceptors. Members of the team share the responsibility for clinical learning. Clinical nurses assist individual students in the nursing care of patients on their unit, being both coach and mentor. Faculty members interact with students and preceptors, linking clinical and classroom learning. Within the model, faculty members unfamiliar with the model need specific preparation for their role. Through discussion, faculty role components are identified and conceptualized. Faculty members help students to process knowledge in the social context of the clinical experience (Yonge, Ferguson, Myrick, & Haase, 2003). Having a dialog with students during the clinical experience could be a challenge, and faculty learn how to best integrate these important conversations into the clinical day. In seminars, faculty provide feedback as well as a forum for reflection of practice. Faculty also cultivate relationships with preceptors. This is essential to providing a supportive environment for clinical learning and developing preceptors for future classes. The effectiveness of the CPMT depends on the relationship between faculty and clinical nurses working with students. Being teamed with a preceptor allows students more time to participate in direct patient care, as opposed to the traditional clinical model of 10 students with one faculty, in which students often spend more time waiting for faculty than actually delivering care (Schreier et al., 2009).

The CPMT model offers several advantages. Students rapidly learn clinical routines. There are increased opportunities to practice skills and to care for multiple patients. When students are paired with unit nurses, there are multiple opportunities for observation of professional nurses' communication and assessment skills. Students received immediate feedback for questions and performance. During the experience, students conduct clinical projects using evidence-based practice relevant to their assigned unit and have the opportunity to present projects to unit staff. In this model, there is a collaborative approach between health care organizations and the college of nursing (Schreier et al., 2009).

Student-Centered Active Teaching Strategies to Meet Learning Needs

There are various recommended learner-centered instructional pedagogies to meet the learning need of students in accelerated programs. For instance, case-based learning is the primary teaching method used to facilitate learning when using instructional technology in the classroom (Morgan Cleave-Hogg, Desousa, & Lam-McCulloch, 2006).

Using human patient simulators are other student-centered approaches frequently used in nursing education and training programs as a means of supplementing clinical experiences for nursing students, reinforcing the use of evidence-based research for practicing nurses, and to enhance the clinical decision-making abilities of the practitioner (Lasater, 2007). High-fidelity patient simulators are becoming an increasingly popular instructional tool for training nurses in acute care settings. This type of instructional technology offers a wide range of interactive and experiential learning opportunities that mimic real-life clinical situations, and allows the learner to analyze, synthesize, apply, infer, evaluate, and compare information that may enhance nurses' critical thinking and the quality of their nursing practice (Kaddoura, 2010). Table 2.1 provides a summary of the curricular innovation and future directions of accelerated nursing programs.

CONCLUSION

Curriculum development, ongoing evaluation, and redesigning are essential activities for nursing faculty. Determining how to best facilitate the learning process, working together as a team to identify and overcome potential challenges embedded in any nursing faculty, and being innovative to meet the challenges of educating future generations of competent nurses are key elements for successful curriculum development or redesign. Ongoing challenges of the increasing volume of information in nursing, the trend toward developing interdisciplinary curricula, the faculty-student gap in today's technologically savvy environment, and meeting the requirements of regulatory agencies are all important issues to address in developing nursing curricula for the 21st century. Baccalaureate Nursing curricula need to be radically changed to incorporate innovative educational models that result in improved students' learning.

The future of accelerated programs is extremely promising. The success of accelerated programs is contingent upon well-designed curricula, qualified nursing faculty, innovation, and adequate resources. Best practice for accelerated nursing education necessitates an understanding of each student's individual learning needs and an understanding of how best to support students in the context of their adult lives. Accelerated students appreciate a variety of active teaching and learning strategies such as the case study teaching approach. Therefore, colleges that offer accelerated nursing programs need to consider how best to prepare faculty to teach these students, who bring new ways of viewing the nursing profession and the health care system overall.

REFERENCES

American Association of Colleges of Nursing. (2008). *The essentials of baccalaureate education for professional nursing practice*. Retrieved from www.aacn.nche.edu/Education/pdf/BaccEssentials08.pdf

American Association of Colleges of Nursing. (2009, September 28). *Nursing Shortage Fact Sheet*. Retrieved from http://www.lchc.org/research/documents/NrsgShortageFS.pdf.

American Association of Colleges of Nursing. (2010). *Fact sheet: Nursing shortage*. Retrieved from http://www.aacn.nche.edu/media/factsheets/nursingshortage.htm

American Nurses Association. (2004). *Nursing: Scope and standards of practice* (4th ed.). Silver Spring, MD: Author.

Beal, J. A. (2007). Accelerated baccalaureate programs: What we know and what we need to know: Setting a research agenda. *Journal of Nursing Education, 46*(9), 387-8.

Bellack, J. P. (2008). Letting go of the rock. *Journal of Nursing Education, 47*(10), 439-440.

Bradshaw, M. J., & Lowenstein, A. J. (2010). *Innovative teaching strategies in nursing and related health professions* (5th ed.). Sunbury, MA: Jones & Bartlett.

Candela, L., Dalley, K., & Benzel-Lindley, J. (2006). A case for learner-centered curricula. *Journal of Nursing Education, 45*(2), 59-66.

Cangelosi, P. (2007). Voices of graduates from second-degree baccalaureate nursing programs. *Journal of Professional Nursing, 23*, 97.

Cangelosi, P. R., & Whitt, K. J. (2005). Accelerated nursing programs: What do we know? *Nursing Education Perspectives, 26*, 113-116.

Connor, C. (2003). Evaluating web-supported learning verses lecture-based teaching: Quantitative and qualitative perspectives. *Innovations in Education and Teaching International, 40*(4), 341-347.

Coonan, P. R. (2008). Educational innovation: Nursing's leadership challenge. *Nursing Economics, 26*(2), 117-122.

Crone, I., & MacKay, K. (2007). Motivating today's college students. *Association of American Colleges and Universities: Peer Review, 9*(1), 18-21.

Cronenwett, L., Sherwood, B., Barnsteiner, J., Disch, J., Johnson, J., Mitchell, P. et al. (2007). Quality and safety education for nurses. *Nursing Outlook, 55*(3), 122-131.

Domrose, C. (2001). You can go home again. *Nurse Week, 1*, 13-14.

Dreher, H. M. (2008). Innovation in nursing education: Preparing for the future of nursing practice. *Holistic Nursing Practice, 22*(2), 77-80.

Ebbertt, D., & Connors, H. (2004). Standardized patient experiences: Evaluation of clinical performance and nurse practitioner student satisfaction. *Nursing Education Perspective, 25*(1), 12-15.

Ferguson, L., & Day, R. A. (2005). Evidence-based nursing education: Myth or reality? *Journal of Nursing Education, 44*(3), 107-115.

Glasgow, M. E., & Cornelius, F. H. (2005). Benefits and costs of integrating technology into undergraduate nursing programs. *Nursing Leadership Forum, 9*, 175-179.

Glennon, C. (2006). Reconceptualizing program outcomes. *Journal of Nursing Education, 45*(2), 5559.

Goodin, H. J., & Stein, D. (2008). Deliberate discussion as an innovative teaching strategy. *Journal of Nursing Education, 47*(6), 272-274.

Hargreaves, J. (2008). Risk: the ethics of a creative curriculum. *Innovations in Education and Teaching International, 45*(3), 227-234.

Hartman, J. L., Dziuban, C., & Brophy-Ellison, J. (2007). Faculty 2.0. EDUCAUSE review, *42*(5), 62-76. Retrieved from http://www.educause.edu/apps/er/erm07/erm0753.asp

Institute of Medicine. (2010). *The future of nursing: Leading change, advancing health*. Washington, DC: Author. Retrieved from http://www.iom.edu/Reports/2010/The-Future-of-Nursing-Leading-Change-Advancing-Health.aspx

Ironside, P., & Valiga, T. M. (2007). How innovative are we? What is the nature of our innovation? *Nursing Education Perspectives, 28*(1), 51-53.

Ironside, P. M.; & Valiga, T. M. (2006). Creating a vision for the future of nursing education: Moving toward excellence through innovation (Guest Editorial). *Nursing Education Perspectives, 27*(3), 120-121.

Iwasiw, C. L., Goldenberg, D., & Andrusyszyn, M. (2009). *Curriculum development in nursing education* (2nd ed.). Sudbury, MA: Jones & Bartlett.

Johnson, J. P., & Mighten, A. (2005) Comparison of teaching strategies: Lecture notes combined with structured group discussion versus lecture only. *Journal of Nursing Education, 44*(7), 319-322.

Kaddoura, M. A. (2010). Perception of clinical simulation on new graduate nurses' critical thinking, learning, and confidence. *The Journal of Continuing Education in Nursing, 41*(11), 506-516.

Lasater, K. (2007). High fidelity simulation and the development of clinical judgment: Student experiences. *Journal of Nursing Education, 46*, 269-276.

Leinonen, P., & Järvelä, S. (2006). Facilitating interpersonal evaluation of knowledge in a context of distributed team collaboration. *British Journal of Educational Technology, 37*(6), 897-916.

Lynch, D. J. (2006). Motivational factors, learning strategies and resource management as predictors of course grades. *The College Student Journal, 40*(2), 423-427.

Melnyk, B. M., & Davidson, S. (2009). Creating a culture of innovation in nursing education through shared vision leadership, interdisciplinary partnerships and positive deviance. *Nursing Administration Quarterly, 33*(4), 288-295.

Morgan, P. J., Cleave-Hogg, D., Desousa, S., & Lam-McCulloch, J. (2006). Applying theory to practice in undergraduate education using high fidelity simulation. *Medical Teacher, 28*, 10-5.

Moscato, S. R., Miller, J., Logsdon, K., Weinberg, S., & Chorpenning, L. (2007). Dedicated education unit: An innovative clinical partner education model. *Nursing Outlook, 55*(1), 31-37.

National Council of State Boards of Nursing. (2009). National Council of State Boards of Nursing: *Transition evidence grid*. Retrieved from https://www.ncsbn.org/Final_08_Transition_grid.pdf

National League for Nursing. (2005). *Transforming nursing education*. [Position Statement]. [Online]. Retrieved from www.nln.org/aboutnln/PositionStatements/transforming052005.pdf.

Pardue, K. T., Tagliareni, M. E., Valiga, T., Davison-Price, M., & Orchowsky, S. (2005). Substantive innovation in nursing education: Shifting the emphasis from content coverage to student learning. *Nursing Education Perspectives, 26*(1), 55-57.

Raines, C. F. (2010). *The doctor of nursing practice: A report on progress*. Paper presented at AACN Spring Annual Meeting.

Reese, C. E., Jeffries, P. R., & Engun, S. A. (2010). Using simulation to develop nursing and medical student collaboration. *Nursing Education Perspectives, 31*(1), 33–37.

Schreier, A. M., Peery, A., & McLean, C. (2009). An integrative curriculum for accelerated nursing education programs. *Journal of Nursing Education, 48,* 282–285.

Schunk, D. (2004). *Learning Theories: An Educational Perspective* (4th ed.). New York: Prentice-Hall.

Shiber, S. (2003). A nursing education model *for second-degree students. Nursing Education Perspectives, 24*(3), 135–138.

Spunt, D., Dawn, M., & Adams, K. (2004). Mock code: A clinical simulation module. *Nurse Educator, 29*(50), 192–194.

Suplee, P. D., & Glasgow, M. E. (2008). Curriculum innovation in an accelerated BSN program: The ACE model. *International Journal of Nursing Education Scholarship, 5*(1), 1.

Tanner, C. A. (2008). Clinical judgment and evidence-based practice: Toward pedagogies of integration. *Journal of Nursing Education, 47*(8), 335–336.

Williams, J. (2002). Education for genetics and nursing practice. *AACN Clinical Issues Advanced Practice in Acute Critical Care, 13*(4), 492–500.

Yonge, O., Ferguson, L., Myrick, F., & Haase, M. (2003). Faculty preparation for the preceptorship experience: The forgotten link. *Nurse Educator, 28,* 210–211.

Chapter 3

Clinical Immersion as an Innovative Pedagogical Approach in Accelerated BSN Programs

Mahmoud Kaddoura, Terri Jabaley, and Collette Williams

INTRODUCTION

*I*n accelerated nursing education, innovative curriculum shifts away from the traditional model to a pedagogical approach, with a greater urgency in ensuring competency for nursing practice in today's complex health care environment. In the traditional model, didactics are typically delivered alongside clinical experiences. Clinical instructors often find themselves providing impromptu lectures in hospital hallways to students who have not yet learned about particular disease processes or nursing interventions in class. Accelerated curricula contrast this approach, recognizing the need for innovative changes in the delivery and coordination of didactic and clinical. At the national level, responses to the NLN position statement, "Innovation in Nursing Education: A Call to Reform" (National League for Nursing, 2003), have primarily taken the form of changes to curricular content. However, the need for reform of both curricular content and underlying curricular delivery mechanisms is needed (National League for Nursing, 2006).

Nursing curriculum design and delivery over the past forty years has been primarily based on behavioralist theory. Ralph Tyler, a prominent

American educator, published a foundational work in 1969 that heavily influenced curriculum design in education. Tyler introduced principles of curriculum and instruction based on behavioralist theory (Tyler, 1969). Tyler viewed curriculum as a planned and directed activity of the school in attaining its educational goals for students. Tyler advocated clearly defined purposes and objectives. He viewed curriculum as the knowledge, skills, and attitudes to be taught and learned at various levels. His approach to evaluation followed specific steps. Situations in which measurement techniques could be used to evaluate achievement were based on specifically defined goals and objectives. From these goals and objectives, performance could be evaluated (Tyler, 1969). Tyler's approach remains the most common in education. Traditionally, nursing education has been based on Tyler's model, which has remained essentially unchallenged until the present. Recently, a number of problems with this approach to curriculum theory and practice have been recognized. First and foremost, it is primarily faculty focused, giving the student little voice, power, or control over their education. Learners are mostly passive. The curriculum exists prior to the learning experience. The measures of success or failure are predesigned. This results in little opportunity for reflection, adaptability, and change in the learning environment (Schaefer & Zygmont, 2003).

There is a need for a new, innovative approach that is learner centered. The driving forces for reform are both internal and external to nursing. Internal forces are evidenced in guiding documents from national nursing organizations such as the AACN (2008) and the National League for Nursing (2006). Recognition of the need for change also comes from groups that influence health care policy and provision, such as the Joint Commission (2011) and the Institute of Medicine (2010). External demands for nursing education reform are also fueled by changes in the nursing practice environment; the shift of care from institutional to the home and community, the exponential growth of knowledge, the increase in technology, and the increasing complexity and acuity of care. Other forces relate to current health care trends and needs in the United States, such as the increase in chronic illness, an aging population, and the need for greater focus on health promotion. Nursing education also faces internal challenges that affect the need for change. Outdated models of clinical education and the limitation of number and quality of clinical education sites are stressors faced by nursing programs. The education of nursing's future generations depends on curricular transformation that keeps up with the ever changing health care delivery system. These issues call for continued reflection and responsiveness. New models of nursing education have emerged to address the challenge of preparing competent generalist nurses, as the health care environment, the profession of nursing, and the typical nursing student have changed. Clinical education models that are better designed to facilitate quality preparation for nursing graduates are emerging.

The clinical immersion model (CIM) is an innovative approach that responds to the calls for programmatic reforms. This model allows students to be immersed in clinical experience after extensive exposure to the theoretical component of nursing courses. The CIM has shown promise in making more meaningful connections between didactic and clinical. In this chapter, the authors teaching in accelerated programs will present an overview of the CIM and its application in accelerated baccalaureate nursing programs.

The CIM is used in both generic accelerated and second-degree accelerated baccalaureate nursing programs. The intention of the CIM is to help students to bridge gaps between theory and practice and be well prepared for competent clinical practice after graduation. In the CIM, the majority of theoretical content is provided in the first half of each clinical nursing course, a period called front loading. The concept of front loading followed by clinical immersion contrasts with the traditional model of nursing education, where the student is taught theory and enters clinical at the same time. Front loading is similar to the concept of mini-term, where course content is delivered over a shortened period of time with longer, focused time in class each day. During front loading, the didactic portion of class is held for approximately four hours per day for two weeks. During this time, students are exposed to the bulk of didactic content prior to their clinical experience. The theoretical content is composed of coursework and clinical lab experience that includes simulation. The CIM promotes clinical competence through attention to progressive content mastery.

After the front-loading period, the student enters the clinical setting in what is called clinical immersion. Clinical immersion allows the student to spend a concentrated amount of time in the clinical setting, three to four days per week for five to six weeks. Students submit clinical reflections weekly to clinical faculty and have traditional pre- and post-conference time with clinical faculty. However, in addition to this, during clinical immersion, students return to the classroom for one day per week. This provides a time and place outside of clinical to reflect on what they have learned and practiced, and receive input and guidance from faculty as the course and their clinical experience progresses. The classroom becomes more dynamic during this time. Faculty provide students with opportunities in class to share experiences from clinical, not just with their small clinical group, but with all of their classmates.

Objectives for each course are specific and leveled so that they increase in complexity with each course. Therefore, students are better able to demonstrate competent care in clinical areas as patient care environments change and acuity increases. During clinical immersion, students spend three days per week in clinical areas such as medical–surgical nursing, maternal–child, mental health, community health, and a final capstone experience. The capstone, a preceptorship in the student's chosen area, involves independent learning and real-world experience designed to transition the student to professional practice. Students are held accountable for a high level of clinical preparation. A well-developed laboratory environment is critical to upholding this expectation. All clinical courses are pass/fail, with well-defined clinical behaviors and competencies. Students are expected to develop their clinical skills and knowledge with faculty guidance, and progress in functioning independently.

CHALLENGES

Intensive Theoretical Content Without Application

As mentioned previously, in the traditional model of nursing education, the student is taught theory and enters clinical simultaneously. The clinical environment is complex, sometimes unpredictable or uncertain, with variation in experiences available to students, including patient illnesses and levels of acuity. Quite often, students' clinical experience may or may not match what they have been taught in the classroom that week. Without a comprehensive theoretical foundation of knowledge, it is challenging for clinical instructors to make patient care assignments that are appropriate to students' level of knowledge, and to support students when clinical situations are reflective of theory that has not yet been learned. This problem is compounded by the fact that in acute care settings, most patients have multiple health problems that need to be assessed, cared for, and evaluated simultaneously.

The organization of theoretical content learned in the classroom and the application of this content in clinical situations present major challenges to nursing faculty. Within the CIM, front loading and clinical immersion must exist together in each clinical nursing course. This design is not without limitations. The concentrated amount of time spent in the classroom is demanding for both students and faculty. Faculty must be highly skilled in providing an environment that is active and conducive to learning. The delivery of material through traditional lecture alone is not sufficient. Student evaluations reveal that it is challenging to maintain attention for lengthy classes, and they often request that diverse, active teaching methods be employed in the classroom. Faculty are challenged to engage students and to remain fresh and interactive themselves throughout class time. Additionally, during the front-loading period, students have no clinical experience to draw upon to apply to the knowledge they are learning in the classroom. Therefore, the faculty are not able to pull upon students' clinical experiences to enhance classroom discussion during the front-loading period. Students are often eager to begin clinical, because it is at this time that information begins to make sense and learning objectives are achieved. This can be beneficial in motivating students to fully apply themselves when clinical experiences begin, or it can be a limitation for students who are primarily affective and kinesthetic learners, who have a greater need for application in order to synthesize knowledge.

Integration of the Essentials of Baccalaureate Education for Professional Nursing Practice

Health care delivery has changed dramatically since the Essentials of Baccalaureate Education for Professional Nursing Practice were first sanctioned by the American Association of Colleges of Nursing (AACN) in 2008 (American Association of Colleges of Nursing, 2008). Building a safer health care system has become the focus of all health care professions, including nursing, following the release of reports from health care authorities such as the Institute of Medicine (2010), the American Hospital Association (2009), the Robert Wood Johnson Foundation (Kimball & O'Neill, 2002), and the Joint Commission (2011). Nursing has been identified as having the potential for making the largest impact on a transformation of health care delivery to a safer, higher-quality, and more cost-effective system (Nelson, Batalden, & Godfrey, 2007).

The AACN Essentials for Baccalaureate Education for Professional Nursing Practice (2008) were developed in response to calls for reform in preparing baccalaureate nurses for the continuously changing health care environment. These recommendations provide a framework for achieving specific outcomes of nursing graduates and emphasize patient-centered care, interprofessional teamwork, evidence-based practice, quality improvement, patient safety, informatics, clinical reasoning/critical thinking, genetics and genomics, cultural sensitivity, professionalism, and practice across the lifespan. The essentials guide nursing educators to develop learning experiences sufficient in breadth and depth to adequately prepare the nursing graduate for entry into today's complex health care arena. Clinical experiences are critical to this preparation. The essentials point to clinical immersion as an effective means for building clinical reasoning, management, and evaluation skills.

The traditional clinical teaching model has not incorporated in depth and breadth the AACN's *Essentials of Baccalaureate Education for Professional Nursing Practice* (2008) to ensure that nursing graduates attain practice-focused outcomes; that is, the knowledge and skills to manage patient-centered care as part of an interprofessional team. Students often have limited interaction with professionals and limited participation in carrying out leadership and management skills within the clinical setting. Students often consider themselves to be outsiders, and nursing staff do not consider them to be part of the professional team within a clinical setting. Although self-reflection is a valuable tool used by nursing faculty in evaluating clinical performance, the need for well-designed clinical experiences based on a broader foundation of knowledge with greater immersion in the professional environment is needed.

The CIM provides intensive, focused clinical opportunities for students to experience some of the key issues referenced in the essentials. For example, clinical immersion incorporates quality and safety issues in the clinical experience, with leveled objectives from the first through the capstone experience. Focused leadership skill development is an integral part of the clinical experience of students in the preceptorship experience. Weekly clinical conferences are dedicated to preparing students for leadership roles and management functions based on their clinical experiences.

It is challenging to fully incorporate AACN Essential 4 [Information Management and Application of Patient Care Technology] in the clinical learning experience. There is often not enough orientation time or synchronous clinical time for students to fully master informatics skills as well as technology used at the bedside. Students often go to various environments for clinical learning and struggle to master the technology specific to each health care system. In the CIM, students' immersion, with focused clinical time, allows better mastery of the concepts essential to information management and use of technology in health care. The concentrated time spent promotes sufficient mastery of the system and time to focus on principles of information management as well.

Additional challenges have been faced to incorporate AACN Essential 6 [Interprofessional Communication and Collaboration for Improving Patient Health Outcomes] and Essential 8 [Professionalism and Professional Values]. Students often enter the initial clinical course with little confidence in their ability to communicate professionally and effectively with patients and other providers, such as physicians.

Clinical experiences are often fragmented in the traditional model, due to the attempt to incorporate clinical time into didactic presentation time. The CIM presents a new approach. To be most effective in preparing students for nursing practice, clinical immersion should be used early in the curriculum. Intensive experiences, conducted after extensive exposure to a theoretical foundation in each course and designed to address course objectives, are imperative. This allows the student to more fully develop generalist knowledge and skills.

Enhancing Critical Thinking and Lifelong Learning

Critical thinking is a crucial outcome of nursing educational programs. Nurse educators are obliged to provide students with learning opportunities that challenge them to think critically in order to solve clinical problems and provide safe and quality care. Another challenge for nursing faculty is to prepare students to be accountable for their own learning and to be lifelong learners. In clinical settings, students need to be provided with opportunities for professional communication and socialization. The CIM offers intensive clinical teaching that establishes a base for more independent nursing roles, especially in the final two semesters of the program. Using clinical immersion allows students to translate their learned theory in various clinical settings such as community health, acute care, and critical care. Through the CIM, students possess a broader knowledge base as they enter the clinical arena, which better prepares them to make good clinical judgments and develop critical thinking skills. Another expected outcome of the CIM is to provide opportunities for students to become engaged with staff nurses and to experience the clinical operations of the nursing unit for three full shifts per week. Although a consistent and extended patient assignment is ideal for novice learners, such opportunities are rarely possible in acute care environments because of rapid patient turnover. The intensive clinical exposure allows students to experience the critical thinking required to respond to evolving situations and to see the value of continuity of care. Within the CIM, students witness rapid shifts in patient populations and conditions. They may care for four or five different patients a week as their assigned patients are admitted and discharged. The experience is reflective of the current reality of nursing and the health care system. Table 3.1 provides a summary of the clinical immersion challenges of accelerated nursing programs.

TABLE 3.1 Summary of Challenges, Strategies, and Future Directions for Clinical Immersion

CHALLENGES	STRATEGIES	FUTURE DIRECTIONS
Intensive theoretical content without application	Application of the clinical immersion model in generic and second-degree accelerated nursing curricula	Recommendations for future accelerated nursing education using the CIM
Integration of the Essentials of Baccalaureate Education for Professional Nursing Practice	Innovative clinical teaching	Bridging the theory practice gap with clinical simulation
Enhancing critical thinking and lifelong learning	Competency measures Development and evaluation	Integration of the AACN's Baccalaureate Nursing Education Essentials
	Student self-evaluation	Continuing the development of students' critical thinking
	Application of critical thinking Preparing students for the licensure exam	

STRATEGIES

Clinical Immersion Model in Generic and Second-Degree Accelerated Nursing Curricula

Student evaluations and learning outcomes have demonstrated that multiple teaching and learning methods are important for faculty to use in the CIM. During front loading, faculty are challenged to collaborate with students in creating an effective learning environment. To address this challenge, active learning in the classroom, such as the use of case studies, games, problem-based scenarios, clickers or other interactive technology, student-to-student interaction, and group work are imperative. Preparation for these classes is time intensive but critical to ensuring student engagement and active learning. Providing adequate support for faculty during the front-loading period can be challenging. Intensive resources are needed. Providing adequate time not only for class preparation and support in collaborative teaching, but also for assistance with test construction and grading of assignments during this intensive time puts a strain on faculty resources. Faculty must be experienced and skilled at bringing the information alive in the classroom for learning to occur, but if planned well, can result in a student who is well prepared for a clinical rotation.

When entering the clinical setting, the student has a more comprehensive knowledge base that he or she can apply in the clinical setting, as opposed to beginning clinical practice with gaps in theoretical knowledge needed for application. With a front-loading approach, the student is better prepared to be fully immersed in the reality of health care delivery, where patient care has become more complex, mirroring the reality that people's health issues are more complex.

In an accelerated baccalaureate curriculum, students spent a considerable amount of time in the nursing laboratory in preparation for the clinical environment. Beginning in fundamentals, students learn and practice basic nursing skills. The lab experience becomes more complex as students progress through clinical courses. Laboratory experiences are carefully planned to progress the student from simple to complex clinical scenarios, using low- and high-fidelity simulation, matched to specific application objectives for students. Individual evaluation and remediation planning are key to a successful lab experience. Open laboratory time is important for students who need remediation. Attention to and documentation of individual students' needs for remediation is an important faculty responsibility. Some of the clinical courses provide a period of skills review called "skills blitz." Here, students are exposed to a review of selected skills specific to the respective course before entering the clinical arena. The faculty provide guidance and evaluation during this time, with additional open lab hours for remediation as necessary, or additional practice in preparation for clinical. Student evaluations reveal that one of the benefits of skills blitz simulation is the increased level of confidence they acquire as they master skills in simulation. Students want complex scenario-based simulation in preparation for real patient care. Faculty strives to formulate simulation experiences that are as realistic as possible, and the approach to clinical skills in the lab is taken seriously by both faculty and students.

With clinical immersion, the student is exposed to a comprehensive base of theoretical content and given the opportunity to practice clinical skills prior to entering the "real" clinical environment, where they will interact directly with patients and use their knowledge and skills to deliver nursing care. In the clinical immersion model, the clinical faculty has a more liberal choice of assignments because the student's knowledge base is broader and more comprehensive when they enter clinical practicum.

Innovative Clinical Teaching

The clinical immersion model is a response to the call for substantive change in the way that nursing students are educated, and a means for integrating the core components of the *Essentials of Baccalaureate Education for Professional Nursing Practice* (American Association of Colleges of Nursing, 2008) into the curriculum. Clinical immersion is a component of all clinical courses, including medical, surgical, maternal, pediatric, mental health, and community health courses. Students who excel also have the opportunity to be chosen for an individual preceptorship with a baccalaureate-prepared RN in a selected setting. In a preceptorship, the student works one-on-one with a preceptor with the oversight of an MSN or higher-degree-prepared nursing faculty. Students are fully immersed in the setting four days per week for the final five to six weeks of their final medical surgical nursing course.

The focused time spent in each of the clinical settings, whether in a clinical group or preceptorship, allows for a less-fragmented, more realistic experience, in which the student has opportunities for participation in leadership development activities, quality improvement projects, and safety initiatives appropriate to the clinical setting. Due to the more consistent presence of students in the clinical setting, clinical staff come to know students better, involving them in operational activities, and integrating them more fully into the health care team. Students also become more proficient in the application and evaluation of technology, through the use of electronic medical and health records, patient monitoring systems, and medication administration systems. They experience, to a greater degree, the reality of professional practice, being more an integrative part of the setting in which they are learning, for a focused, intensive period of time. Students develop a capstone project during their final clinical rotation. This is based on the students' needs assessment of a particular setting, and may include the development or revision of a policy, provision of a community service project, development of a patient or staff education program, or design of a quality improvement program.

Competency Measures Development and Evaluation

Competency development for nursing students occurs through the CIM in a sequential manner, by building competency from simple to complex. Theoretical content provides a foundation for attainment of specific competency outcomes and is sequenced to progress through each course and across the BSN curriculum. Students are exposed to necessary knowledge first via lecture, group discussion, case studies, and problem-solving methods in the front-loaded didactic component of each course. Students are evaluated through quizzes and testing, case study contributions, participation in problem solving, and feedback through the use of clickers or other technologies in the classroom. Learning is enhanced through application of knowledge in the clinical laboratory, where simulations are designed to evaluate students' ability to apply knowledge and to help them develop clinical reasoning in a risk-free environment, where faculty provide individualized guidance and evaluation, remediation, and opportunity for practice and development of students' confidence.

Students then enter the clinical arena with a strong foundation of knowledge and skills, a sense of confidence in their ability to make safe clinical judgments, and the support of faculty who have mentored them through simulated experiences. It is within clinical immersion that the student must be critically evaluated and guided to achieve specific competencies that constitute safe and effective nursing practice. Clinical faculty have specifically defined competencies for each clinical experience and evaluation data from course faculty and laboratory simulations that help them prepare for each clinical student, aware of strengths and weaknesses so that individual plans for the achievement of competency outcomes can be formulated. Communication between course coordinators, classroom faculty, lab faculty, and clinical instructors is imperative to ensure students' seamless transition from didactic learning to clinical learning. Detailed evaluations and areas of concern are communicated to clinical faculty so that they can better develop a plan of success for each student.

Clinical instructors evaluate students on a day-to-day basis in the clinical setting through direct observation, supervision, and specific clinical assignments. Some of the core means of competency evaluation include review of concept maps and plans of care, review of reflective journals, review of clinical decision making, and direct observation of clinical activities such as giving a complete nursing report, performing complete and focused nursing assessments, preparing and delivering medications safely, teaching, and engaging in leadership and management activities. The clinical faculty's observation and evaluation of specific competencies must be comprehensive and consistent among clinical groups within each course. The intensive time in clinical allows faculty to fully evaluate each student within a given week, focusing on the individual student's needs and objectives. Clinical faculty encourage students to self-evaluate, taking time each day to reflect on their practice, plan for improvement for the upcoming day, and thus contribute to their plan for success.

Preceptors evaluate students with the guidance of course objectives and expected clinical outcomes. Core faculty, providing oversight of clinical preceptorships, need to be attentive to both preceptors' and students' ongoing needs. Preceptors have core faculty guidance as needed to provide competency evaluation to the faculty's level of expectancy for the successful evaluation of a student in the course.

Student Self-Evaluation

Students self-evaluate through clinical reflection and are guided to reflect on their own performance as well as patient outcomes. Specific, individual goals must be set at least weekly or at more frequent intervals as necessary with faculty guidance. Constructive feedback from faculty, clinical staff, and patients is consistently communicated to the student through faculty for self-reflection. Allowing students to evaluate their peers can also be helpful in developing clinical decision making and applying clinical skills. Peer and self-evaluation allows the student to focus on areas of weakness and strength that present as they face clinical decisions and apply clinical skills. Multiple forms of constructive feedback help the student to improve upon weaknesses and transform the challenges to opportunities for success. One effective strategy for this evaluation is pairing up students who have alternate strengths and weaknesses, allowing them to give feedback to each other in performing nursing assessment, giving reports, communicating with patients, and making various clinical decisions. The clinical faculty is a facilitator of this ongoing dynamic environment of competency development and serves to clarify, correct, and guide students to find answers as a team. Encouraging positive reinforcement and teamwork among peer students in a clinical group promotes confidence and collegiality. It is helpful in promoting a sense of professionalism and accomplishment important in professional practice. Students learn the value of teamwork, along with methods and skills for multidisciplinary team building that are elements of successful care provision in today's health care settings. Another successful strategy for competency development and evaluation is the recording and reviewing of audio-taped verbal reports. This can be done throughout the clinical day and reviewed by the group at clinical conference or in pairs of students with clinical faculty guidance. Reports at both the hand-off of patient care and use of the situation, background, assessment, and recommendation (SBAR) method for interprofessional communication are evaluated for competency.

Application of Critical Thinking

Through immersion on a clinical nursing unit, the CIM rapidly intro-
duces students to the critical thinking skills necessary for patient care
and provides an enhanced opportunity for professional identification
and socialization. Moreover, intensive clinical experience establishes a
base for more autonomous nursing roles in the final two semesters of
the program, when students take theory and clinical courses in community health, mental health, geriatric care, and advanced adult care with a
leadership focus. The intensive clinical exposure allows students to
experience the critical thinking required to respond to evolving situations and to witness rapid shifts in the patient population. During the
clinical immersion, students may care for four or five different patients
a week as their assigned patients are admitted and discharged. The
experience reflects the current reality of nursing and the health
care system.

Teaching strategies to address accelerated adult learners to foster their
critical thinking consist of state-of-the-art methods such as simulations,
interactive technologies, contemporary topics, clinical concept and
mind mapping, and case-based problem solving. Other active teaching
strategies that can develop accelerated students' critical thinking
include the use of case studies that help learners actually use their
thought process to think independently and collaboratively through the
case to analyze, synthesize, and evaluate the scenario in order to infer
sound clinical judgment (Kaddoura & Williams, 2011). Another strategy
is the use of Socratic questions to help students strengthen their verbal
presentation skills to peers, faculty, and others on the health care team.
The Socratic questions method actively involves students within the
classroom with the expectations of preparation for class. Guided
questioning is a helpful teaching strategy for accelerated students to
think critically through the challenging questions. The faculty can encourage the students to think critically by presenting to them a case and
having them answer, then asking higher-level questions. The goal of
asking higher-level questions is to help students analyze, synthesize, evaluate, and use reasoning skills not only to infer appropriate answers but also
to be able to apply the content in clinical practice (Kaddoura & Williams,
2011). The need for critical-thinking students is also resonating from the
employer arena (Giddens & Brady, 2007). Students will only develop
these skills through a combination of learning experiences derived from
independent, evidence-based practice methods and exposure to experienced faculty and clinicians. The persistence of faculty in teaching

excessive content within inadequate timeframes is counterproductive to the development of critical thinking skills and remains an unresolved issue (Zygmont & Schaeffer, 2006).

Preparing Students for the Licensure Exam

From the beginning of an accelerated BSN nursing program, students are immersed in a culture of NCLEX-RN success. Philosophical tenets of the NCLEX-RN culture build the reflective practice model elements that challenge faculty and students to reflect on actions, assess outcomes, and seek ongoing improvement (Walker et al., 2007). Because the NCLEX-RN is based on the concepts of critical thinking, analysis, synthesis, inference, evaluation, and reasoning, the accelerated nursing students incorporate these concepts into their course through adopting the NCLEX test plan developed by the National Council of States Boards of Nursing (NCSBN, 2009). This plan assumes that as culture is transmitted to new generations, a system of values, beliefs, and traditions that promote NCLEX-RN success can be transmitted to nursing students. Communicating this expectation to think critically in order to pass the NCLEX in a positive and proactive manner removes the punitive signals often perceived by students with regard to remediation activities and the additional efforts required outside of class to ensure success. Accelerated BSN students are considered self-directed learners and have greater expectation for faculty guidance (Walker et al., 2007). The plan challenges the students and faculty to reflect on testing progress and take action for remediation toward improving NCLEX-RN outcomes through enhancing the critical thinking skills of accelerated nursing students. Teaching strategies that stimulate critical thinking are incorporated into the courses of the accelerated nursing programs. Some strategies that facilitate the process include concept mapping, games, student-generated test items, and assessment tests based on readings. A majority of these activities can be accomplished by student teams in case-based learning and problem-based learning strategies of teaching. Critical thinking skills of accelerated second-degree nursing students are significantly higher than those of traditional nursing students ($p = 0.017$), supporting the ability of second-degree students to quickly assimilate new knowledge related to nursing practice and progress through a nursing program at an accelerated rate (Pepa, Brown, & Alverson, 1997). Table 3.1 provides a summary of the clinical immersion strategies of accelerated nursing programs.

FUTURE DIRECTIONS

Recommendations for Future Accelerated Nursing Education Using the CIM

Many lessons have been learned through application of the CIM. As noted earlier, the initial front-loading period in the CIM is demanding for both students and faculty. Students must be prepared for the intensive nature of learning during this time. The expectation for them to commit to the required reading and preparation for each day of class should be clearly articulated. Faculty must maintain competency in conducting lengthy classes, providing adequate break time, and maximizing the use of teaching and learning techniques in the classroom. Faculty workload during this time should be considered, and management has a responsibility to lessen meeting time and other program requirements for faculty during the two-week front-loading process. Teamwork and communication among faculty is imperative, as the learning and evaluation process progresses from simple to complex in classroom, lab, and clinical. Students are unable to progress to more complex implementation of knowledge and skills if they have not mastered the basics. Attention to student progress in meeting objectives is imperative among faculty. Regular meetings and tools to promote effective communication from course to course are essential. Communication needs to be streamlined, accessible, and useful among faculty in order to provide an accurate and fair competency evaluation and remediation process for each student with his or her unique strengths and weaknesses. Clinical faculty are in a critical role for assuring that students have not only mastered content in their minds, but are also able to put into practice what they have learned in a safe and effective way. Therefore, managers are challenged to secure appropriate settings and competent clinical faculty. Core faculty should also realize the importance of constant communication and follow-up with clinical faculty and students during clinical immersion to ensure adequate competency development.

Bridge the Theory–Practice Gap With Clinical Simulation

Simulations are a valuable tool in nursing education, providing a bridge from theory to application in clinical practice. They are becoming the cornerstone of a comprehensive laboratory experience that provides nursing students with a safe, realistic practice arena for growth in competence and confidence. Simulation is an essential component of the CIM in preparing students for clinical interaction with actual patients. Simulation provides faculty with the opportunity for evaluation and remediation of students' proficiency in clinical decision making in an environment that is confidential and proposes no risk to an actual patient. In well-constructed simulation, the student experiences a sense of reality, yet is aware that they cannot hurt the patient, allowing them more autonomy in making decisions that otherwise would involve risks to actual patients. Simulated experiences can be leveled from simple to complex to facilitate students' progress in meeting objectives through the nursing curriculum. High-fidelity simulation provides the opportunity for students to make clinical judgments and practice interventions in common clinical situations or unusual emergent situations, chosen by the faculty to meet specific course objectives. Simulation experience accelerates expertise and can help facilitate the path from novice to expert, which otherwise occurs more slowly through actual clinical experience (Jeffries, 2007).

To help bridge the gap between theory and practice, comprehensive lab experiences followed by collaboration with a variety of health care facilities for provision of rich clinical experiences for students is imperative. The lab experience should bridge the gap between classroom and clinical. Comprehensive lab preparation is key to the students' successful transition. A technologically current lab environment along with an updated pedagogy for students' transition from classroom to clinical is needed. Comprehensive lab activities should begin early in the program, during the first semester. Faculty should orient students to the lab and simulation manikins and allow students to practice basic skills and become familiar with much of the equipment they will encounter throughout the program. Low-fidelity simulation practice should be implemented for basic skills practice and progressively advanced to integrate high-fidelity simulation as appropriate throughout the curriculum.

Readings, skills CDs, and lab equipment are important resources for students' learning. Students entering the senior-year clinical immersion demonstrate competency in prior learned skills via simulation case studies and virtual clinical experiences. Students are presented case studies, asked to perform skills and assessments on the simulation manikins, and answer questions related to critical thinking, problem solving, and clinical decision making. The real-life scenarios and case studies, both faculty-developed and commercially available virtual clinical experiences, ensure competence and confidence when entering the clinical settings.

In addition to comprehensive state of the art lab preparation, students are required to be engaged in field experiences during the theoretical component of the model. Most nursing courses during the first year of the accelerated BSN program have a specific set of clinical field experiences ranging from one to six hours each. These are used to meet course objectives and reinforce class content such as observations of community, for example, homeless population in shelters, prisoners, nursing home residents, and hospice. They may also include mandatory flu clinics as part of community service learning. Other field experiences may include observations in labor and delivery, the operating room, the postanesthesia care unit, radiology, special procedures such as gastro-intestinal lab (endoscopy, colonoscopy), pulmonary lab (bronchoscopy), kidney dialysis, or with school nurses and hospital specialty nurses, providing real-life contact with patients and the ability to observe and model professional nursing behaviors to reinforce class-related concepts. Field experiences are set up by faculty and are required of students, but they are completed like homework outside scheduled class time. They are remotely supervised by faculty and directly supervised by designees of the clinical agencies, such as staff nurses. The shift of the responsibility for completing field experiences to the student enhances students' accountability for their own learning. To evaluate field experiences, students are required to reflect on their experiential learning and maintain reflective journals. Such short-written assignments help promote students' reflective learning and documentation competency. Part of the success of the clinical immersion model relies on faculty holding students accountable for the sum of their educational experiences to the point of the final clinical immersion year.

Integration of the AACN's Baccalaureate Nursing Education Essentials

The nine AACN Essentials are crucial curricular elements that should provide the framework for accelerated baccalaureate clinical nursing edu-cation. In each nursing course, faculty are required to emphasize basic concepts of liberal education [Essential 1]. In order to prepare the bacca-laureate nursing student for generalist nursing practice, continuing the pedagogical approach of intensive, reflective writing assignments to promote reflection, insight, and integration of ideas across disciplines and courses helps students to develop intellectual and innovative capacities for current and developing generalist nursing practice.

Organizational and systems leadership, quality improvement, and patient safety [Essential 2] are crucial to providing high-quality patient care. Innovative clinical models should incorporate leadership skills that emphasize ethical and clinical decision making, initiating and maintaining effective working relationships, using mutually respectful communication and collaboration within interpersonal teams, care coordination, delegation, and developing conflict resolution strategies. It is recommended that fundamental skills, such as therapeutic communication, interviewing, and health assessment, be developed early in the program. These foundational skills can be practiced along with basic skills such as vital signs, hygiene, and transfers through simulation and field experience.

Students may also be assigned to spend a clinical day with nurse managers to get acquainted with basic nursing leadership skills. Such field visits and observation experiences help raise students' awareness of complex systems and the impact of power, politics, and guidelines on the ever changing health care system. Students would better develop leadership skills through clinical immersion by spending time with nurse leaders. This time would be valuable in developing the student's knowledge and experience with concepts and practices of leadership, healthcare policy, finance, and regulatory environments [Essential 5], all of which are essential concepts for professional nursing practice. Students acquainted with these concepts will possess valuable knowledge to be more attentive to the delivery of cost-effective care and the judicious use of available resources in the health care organization. Scholarship for evidence-based practice [Essential 3] should be integrated within an innovative clinical teaching model. Students should be able to identify current practice issues, appraise and incorporate evidence in their practice, and evaluate outcomes to ensure quality and safety of patient care.

Incorporation of informatics [Essential 4] competencies should be included in the curriculum. Knowledge and skills in information and patient care technology are crucial in preparing nursing graduates to provide quality patient care in a variety of health care settings. In one accelerated BSN program, an informatics course assists students in the process of evaluating health care information on the internet, focusing students on quality of care and safety issues, and providing the history, trends, and future of informatics in nursing. This course runs concurrently with other clinical courses, so that students have the opportunity to reflect on principles of informatics while in the clinical setting.

Nursing faculty members are challenged to educate nursing students to deliver patient-centered care as members in an interprofessional team. Innovative clinical models should provide students with adequate opportunities to apply effective communication and collaboration [Essential 6] among health care professionals as early in the curriculum as possible. Through the CIM, students should be exposed to community settings earlier, so that health promotion and disease prevention are addressed and incorporated throughout clinical experiences. Such exposure would enhance students' professionalism [Essential 8] and prepare them to demonstrate professional standards of moral, ethical, and legal conduct. Innovative clinical models should allow students to assume accountability for personal and professional behaviors. This will promote the image of nursing by modeling the professional values and integrating the knowledge, skills, and attitudes of the nursing profession.

Continuing the Development of Students' Critical Thinking

With the increased need for qualified care providers comes the increased need for competency in the workplace. Health care organizations are seeking ways to attract and retain highly qualified nurses who are able to think critically to cope with the various challenges related to advanced technology and more complex health care systems. In health care facilities, nurses are expected to be caring, critical thinkers, and competent practitioners. Schools of nursing need to produce competent bedside nurses ready to care for patients in a complex, changing health care environment. The need for competent practitioners has never been greater than nowadays, considering the fast-paced advances in technology and patient acuity. Bevis and Watson (2000) suggested: "Nursing knowledge and learning processes for the future require much more thought, contemplation and rejection upon the very concepts and phenomena associated with dramatically changing human conditions and life processes" (p. 38). Table 3.1 provides a summary of the clinical immersion future directions of accelerated nursing programs.

CONCLUSION

Overall, clinical immersion provides students with a more intense and comprehensive experience of patient care than the traditional clinical model. Students enter the clinical setting armed with a broad knowledge base that allows them to approach the application of learning to nursing practice in a more comprehensive way. This contrasts traditional clinical models, in which the student may be in the clinical setting for one or two days per week, returning to class in the same week to acquire more knowledge as the course progresses. The clinical environment provides a rich learning experience, where the student participates in the profession and nursing theory becomes real for them. Students and faculty alike have better opportunities for evaluation in the clinical immersion setting, as there is more concentrated time and more experiences to do so. Clinical faculty has less responsibility for providing impromptu lectures in the clinical setting than in the tradition model. Professional staff in clinical settings get to know students well and feel more comfortable interacting and providing feedback as they come to trust students and feel they are a part of their team. At its essence, clinical immersion is a concentrated clinical experience of applying theory to practice, more comprehensively and sequentially than through traditional models of nursing education. It is an approach that addresses the need for better bridging the gap that exists for nursing students between theory and professional practice.

REFERENCES

American Association of Colleges of Nursing. (2008). *The essentials of baccalaureate education for professional nursing practice*. Retrieved from www.aacn.nche.edu/Education/pdf/BaccEssentials08.pdf

American Hospital Association. (2009). *Teaching hospitals: Their impact on patients and the future health care workforce*. Retrieved from http://www.aha.org/aha/trendwatch/2009/twsept2009teaching.pdf

Bevis, E. O., & Watson, J. (2000). *Toward a caring curriculum: A new pedagogy for nursing*. Boston: Jones & Bartlett.

Giddens, J., & Brady, D. (2007). Rescuing nursing education from content saturation: A case for a concept-based curriculum. *Journal of Nursing Education*, *46*(2), 65–9.

Institute of Medicine (2010). *The future of nursing: Leading change, advancing health*. Washington, DC: Author. Retrieved from http://www.iom.edu/Reports/2010/The-Future-of-Nursing-Leading-Change-Advancing-Health.aspx

Jeffries, P. (2007). *Simulation in nursing education: From conceptualization to evaluation*. New York: National League for Nursing.

The Joint Commission (2011). *The 2011 National Patient Safety Goals*. Retrieved from http://www.jointcommission.org/assets/1/6/2011_NPSGs_HAP.pdf

Kaddoura, M. A., & Williams, C. (2011). Comparison of generic accelerated baccalaureate nursing students' critical thinking (CT) skills before and after implementing the case study pedagogical method and correlation between CT and students' age, gender, and GPA. *Educational Research Quarterly* (In press).

Kimball, B., & O'Neil, E. (2002). *Health care's human crisis: The American nursing shortage*. Princeton, NJ: The Robert Wood Johnson Foundation. Retrieved from http://www.rwjf.org/files/publications/other/NursingReport.pdf

National Council of State Boards of Nursing (2009). *Transition evidence grid*. Retrieved from http://www.ncsbn.org/Final_08_Transition_grid.pdf

National League for Nursing. (2003). *Innovation in nursing: A call to reform*. Retrieved from www.nln.org/aboutnln/PositionStatements/innovation082203.pdf.

National League for Nursing, (2006). *Nurse educators 2006: A report of the faculty census survey of RN and graduate programs*. New York: Author.

Nelson, E. C., Batalden, P. B., & Godfrey, M. M. (2007). *Quality by design: A clinical Microsystems approach*. San Francisco, CA: Jossey-Bass.

Pepa, C. A., Brown, J. M., & Alverson, E. M. (1997). A comparison of critical thinking abilities between accelerated and traditional baccalaureate nursing students. *Journal of Nursing Education, 36*(1), 46–48.

Schaefer, K. M., & Zygmont, D. (2003). Analyzing the teaching style of nursing faculty: Does it promote a student-centered or teacher-centered learning environment? *Nursing Education Perspectives, 24*(5), 238–245.

Tyler, R. W. (1969). *Basic principles of curriculum and instruction.* Chicago: The University of Chicago Press.

Walker, J. T., Martin, T. M., Haynie, L., Norwood, A., White, J., & Grant, L. (2007). Preferences for teaching methods in a baccalaureate nursing program: How second-degree and traditional students differ. *Nursing Education Perspectives, 28*(5), 246–250.

Zygmont, D. M., & Schaeffer, K. M. (2006). Assessing the critical thinking skills of faculty: What do the findings mean for nursing education? *Nursing Education Perspectives, 27*(5), 260–268.

Achieving Excellence in Teaching

Alicia Huckstadt

OVERVIEW AND CHALLENGES OF TEACHING EFFECTIVENESS

*T*eaching effectiveness is a complex, multifactorial concept that involves the teaching – learning process between faculty and students and assessment of learning outcomes. The key to effective learning is knowledgeable and insightful educators (Bradshaw & Lowenstein, 2011) and motivated learners. Ideally, both teaching and learning are active, dynamic processes with an emphasis on the learner and learning. Often, the processes extend beyond the subject matter to a personal inter- active relationship between the learner and teacher (Vandeveer & Norton, 2005). Both teacher and learner are actively engaged in discovering and constructing knowledge, a far shift from the previously held beliefs that students are passive receivers of information, memorizing only for an examination, and teachers control the information. Most educators now perceive education as a dynamic interaction between educators and learners with teaching as a complex, deliberate effort to facilitate "student-driven" learning.

However, teaching effectiveness is often unstated and misunderstood. Educators have an ethical responsibility to assess themselves and students with the most appropriate measures possible. Most nursing educators recognize the importance of education and strive to fulfill their roles, but may not be prepared in the development and use of valid assessment measures. The shortage of nursing faculty, especially those with educational expertise and a terminal degree, is well recognized. Schools/colleges of nursing have recruited and hired MSN-prepared nurses to fulfill the role of faculty. These nurse educators often have clinical expertise but are hired in teaching positions with no prior academic teaching experience. As a result, new faculty members may be ill-prepared to manage the complexities of teaching and assessing learner outcomes.

Teaching effectiveness is a critical and integral part of the larger educational program evaluation. Assessment of teaching effectiveness is contingent on the faculty member, parent institution and academic unit's mission and goals, accrediting organizations, and other stakeholders. All components of program evaluation should promote quality improvement. Internal and external factors such as the parent institution, state legislatures, boards of directors, and others may have standards for accountability such as faculty workload and expectations in teaching, as well as other aspects of service and research.

Nursing educators are responsible and accountable for several essentials of evaluation, including student learning and their own teaching practices, as well as course, curriculum, and program effectiveness outcomes (Bourke & Ihrke, 2005). This hefty responsibility and accountability requires considerable knowledge. Evaluation is the process of making judgments about learning and achievement based on careful analysis of assessment data (Oermann & Gaberson, 2009). Predetermined goals or outcomes guide processes to determine effectiveness (Menix, 2007). Included in evaluation is formative evaluation that occurs on an ongoing basis and summative evaluation that occurs at the end of a learning activity or program.

Teaching excellence is an ongoing quest for universities and colleges. Faculty and administrators are looking for ways to increase knowledge about teaching effectiveness (Hativa, Barak, & Simhi, 2001) and better prepare students for graduation and careers. Unfortunately, most university and college faculty gain beliefs and knowledge about what makes a good teacher through trial-and-error, reflection on student ratings, and using self-evaluation. While educational literature reports provide suggestions for "good teachers," few psychometrically sound studies exist.

Findings of one qualitative study by Hativa et al. (2001) suggested that different exemplary teachers achieve effectiveness in very different ways and teachers do not need to excel in all four main dimensions (lesson organization, lesson clarity, making a lesson interesting/engaging, and conducive classroom climate) specified in this study to be effective. These authors concluded that an essential part of preparing faculty members in their teaching role is to increase their knowledge of a wide variety of teaching strategies and how these strategies contribute to the four main dimensions of effective teaching. Knowledge is only one part in preparing teachers to be effective. Teachers often do not receive direct, objective feedback about their teaching effectiveness. Use of nonstandardized evaluations, heavy reliance on a single evaluation source, and inadequate opportunities to improve teaching strategies hamper educators' progress in achieving teaching effectiveness. Lacking constructive evaluation of their teaching, some educators become discouraged and leave academia.

Helping higher-education teachers believe in themselves and their teaching abilities was the focus of an international study (Roche & Marsh, 2000). In this study, feedback from students' evaluations was found to influence the educators' self-concept. For example, educators who received student evaluations of their teaching effectiveness had higher correlations with their own self-concept than those who had not received previous student evaluations. The authors concluded that educators do respond to the feedback they receive in student evaluations and adjust their self-perceptions accordingly. As such, the interaction between the self-concept of educators and student evaluations is an important consideration in working to improve teacher effectiveness. Other studies have identified successful teaching. For their part, Rossetti and Fox (2009) conducted an interpretive analysis of educational philosophies and goal statements from 35 university professors across five disciplines who received Presidential Teaching Awards from a public mid-western university in the United States. Four relevant areas were identified as successful university teaching themes: (1) Presence or "... deeper level of awareness that allows thoughts, feelings, and actions to be known, developed, and harmonized within" (p. 13); (2) Promotion of learning; (3) Teachers as learners; and (4) Enthusiasm. The researchers concluded that the narratives from this study may help define successful teaching across disciplines and offer nursing educators additional perspectives that they had not yet considered.

Tang, Chou, and Chiang (2005) turned their focus on students' perceptions of clinical teachers. A survey of 214 students in two nursing schools in Taiwan found that effective clinical teachers possessed significantly higher scores in four categories: interpersonal relationships, professional competence, personality characteristics, and teaching ability. Large differences between effective and ineffective teachers were found in interpersonal relationships and personality characteristics. The researchers concluded that the educators' attitudes toward students, rather than their professional abilities, were more revealing for differences between effective and ineffective teachers and they recommended that educators strive to express more positive attitudes toward students.

Faculty members have used a wide variety of teaching methods in an effort to provide all students an opportunity to gain knowledge, regardless of students' learning style or preferences, age, gender, content, and other factors influencing the teaching/learning process (Forrest, 2004). Learning styles can be identified and incorporated into teaching methods. An online learning style and strategies resource by Felder and Soloman from North Carolina State University is available at http://www.uncw. edu/cte/soloman_felder.htm. This resource helps identify learning preferences for active and reflective learners, sensing and intuitive learners, visual and verbal learners, and sequential and global learners. While most individuals are not only one type of learner or may vary when they prefer a type, preference can be mild, moderate, or strong. Active learners understand information best by doing and reflective learners prefer to work alone and think about it. Listening to lectures is particularly difficult for active learners. Sensing learners like to learn facts, use well-established methods, and abhor complications, while intuitive learners prefer innovation, discovering possibilities, and relationships. Sensing learners are more likely than intuitive learners to resent examinations or other evaluation on material that has not been explicitly covered in class. Visual learners remember visual images while verbal learners prefer written and spoken explanations. All learners receive more information when presented both verbally and visually. Sequential learners prefer logical, linear steps of information while global learners learn in large jumps without seeing connections. Global learners may have difficulty explaining how they grasped the big picture. Understanding learners' preferences assist educators in designing teaching methods, and thus, developing themselves as more effective educators.

If educators evaluate their own teaching strategies, they may be able to better facilitate learning for their students. The Center for Research on Teaching and Learning, University of Michigan, offers an online resource for further information about teaching strategies http://www.crlt. umich.edu/tstrategies/tsts.php. This website provides guidance for instructors thinking about their own teaching style and its impact on student learning. Resources within the site include links to teaching surveys and inventories, and suggestions for how to use this information to accommodate the learning needs of their students. Another helpful website, Penn State Learning Design Community Hub http://ets.tlt.psu. edu/learningdesign/audience/teachingstyles, offers the following information on assessing four basic teaching styles: (1) Formal Authority: An instructor-centered approach where the instructor feels responsible for providing and controlling the flow of content, which the student is to receive and assimilate. The formal authority figure neither concerns himself or herself with creating a relationship with the student nor believes it to be important for the students to build relationships with each other; (2) Demonstrator or Personal Model: An instructor-centered approach where the instructor demonstrates and models what is expected (skills and processes) and then acts as a coach or guide to assist the students in applying the knowledge. This style encourages student participation and utilizes various learning styles; (3) Facilitator: A student-centered approach where the instructor facilitates and focuses on activities. Responsibility is assigned to the students to take initiative to achieve results for the various tasks. Students who are independent, active, collaborative learners thrive in this environment. Instructors typically design group activities that necessitate active learning, student-to-student collaboration, and problem solving; and (4) Delegator: A student-centered approach whereby the instructor delegates and places much control and responsibility for learning on individuals or groups of students. This type of instructor will often require students to design and implement a complex learning project and will act solely in a consultative role. Students are often asked to work independently or in groups and must be able to effectively work in group situations and manage various interpersonal roles.

Identification of the teaching types is useful for nursing educators wanting to assess their teaching. An online teaching style survey, Grasha-Riechmann, is also available at http://www.longleaf.net/teaching style.html and is helpful in identifying teaching preferences.

The Texas Collaborative for Teaching Excellence http://www.texas-collaborative.org/TSI.htm also provides a self-assessment instrument with feedback on selected preferred teaching styles. The assessment may be useful in determining the type of learners best suited for each teaching style, or suggest ways to alter the teaching style for other types of learners.

Accelerated nursing programs attract different types of learners and present different challenges to educators than traditional programs. In this light, Walker et al. (2007) studied the preferences for teaching methods between second-degree and traditional baccalaureate nursing students. Significant differences were found between the two groups, with second-degree nursing students reporting stronger preferences in three areas: (1) self-directed learning and motivation; (2) higher expectations for classroom structure and guidance from faculty; and (3) obtaining a grade that matters. The authors concluded that second-degree students are different than traditional students in their educational expectations, preferences for teaching methods, and relationship expectations with faculty. These differences provide challenges to nurse educators as they seek learning environments and teaching methodologies for innovative and accelerated models of nursing education.

Schreier, Peery, and McLean (2009) reported how they changed their educational paradigm from traditional pedagogical to a concept student-learning approach in their accelerated nursing education programs. Fast-paced accelerated programs present unique challenges to the educational process. Cangelosi and Whitt (2005) and later Penprase and Koczara (2009) conducted separate reviews of the literature for understanding the experiences of accelerated second-degree nursing students and concluded that these students are highly independent, self-motivated, and learn independently with instruction and guidance. Integrating diverse teaching and learning methods are likely to increase students' success in these programs.

Lockwood, Walker, and Tilley (2009) examined faculty perceptions of the accelerated baccalaureate nursing program in its inaugural year. These authors found that the faculty had to adapt to a newly implemented teaching model, learn to teach a different kind of student, combine accelerated and traditional students, and learn as they progressed. Teaching methods became important as they recognized that accelerated students were more challenging, stronger clinically, and had better writing skills than the traditional students.

Different teaching and learning strategies are needed for the diverse learners in accelerated programs. Suplee and Glasgow (2008) described the curriculum innovation that was implemented at the Drexel University accelerated baccalaureate program titled The Accelerated Career Entry (ACE) model. The program design emphasizes technology, professional socialization, and use of standardized patients. These authors report that the teaching strategies that are used in more traditional nursing programs may not be effective with accelerated programs. Although the profile for accelerated students is not yet well described, they have been reported to be mature, excellent learners who challenge traditional knowledge. However, the researchers of this study cautioned against assuming all accelerated students to be highly motivated, to communicate effectively, able to manage stress, or know how to manage their time. The faculty of this ACE program found many different learners. The faculty described the students as "challenging, entitled, and assertive at times bordering on aggressive" (Suplee & Glasgow, 2008, p. 1). ACE faculty learned to foster creative thinking, share past experiences in discussions, provide time management sessions, include communication techniques, and refer to counseling departments as needed. Kruszewski, Brough, and Killeen (2009) described a successful collaborative model for teaching evidence-based practice in an accelerated second-degree nursing program by sharing teaching and partnering with clinical nurses in implementing the students' projects. This approach for teaching resulted in a high degree of satisfaction for students, faculty, and clinical nurses in partnering agencies. Mullen (2007) tested accelerated second-degree baccalaureate nursing students' use of self-regulating learning strategies to focus, organize, integrate, and retain knowledge from classroom and clinical sources. A comparison between 49 second- and 76 third-semester students enrolled in a three-semester-long program, demonstrated that both second- and third-semester students used the self-regulating learning strategies; however, third-semester students used more of the strategies than the less-experienced second-semester students. Mullen concluded that the self-learning strategy may be helpful to diverse, nontraditional students in accelerated nursing programs and use of the strategy increases with student learning experience. Mullen added the strategy may also be used to assess non-nursing college graduates requesting admission to accelerated BSN programs as a measure of their academic success.

In their qualitative study of a large private college in New England, Rico, Beal, and Davies (2010) identified six best faculty practices for teaching in accelerated nursing programs: (1) recognize students as adult learners; (2) challenge and motivate students; (3) communicate passion for nursing; (4) clinically practice, stay up-to-date, and weave practice experiences into teaching; (5) support students by believing in them and being openly supportive of the accelerated program; and (6) use varied teaching styles. No one single teaching style, including PowerPoint presentations, case studies, case development, verbal presentations, "Socratic method" questioning, was preferred by accelerated students. Instead, these students preferred a variety of styles.

Blending practice and pedagogy was the theme identified from a qualitative study of 19 accelerated second-degree baccalaureate nursing students who had graduated (Cangelosi, 2007). This study explored how the graduates' experiences during school had best prepared them for nursing practice after graduation. The significance of clinical instructors was identified as the major theme. Recognizing the importance of clinical instruction and importance of competent, clinical instructors who are effective teachers determines the success of programs. Clinical instructors help students apply their classroom learning in the clinical setting. Additional challenges face clinical instructors who transform routine incidents into valuable learning experiences for students. Clinical educators are "often required to orient themselves to multiple clinical sites and decipher large amounts of paperwork related to the teaching of the course" (Cangelosi, 2007, p. 403). This workload, compounded with the fast pace of accelerated programs and frequent perceptions that clinical educators do not receive adequate academic status, presents additional challenges. Cangelosi reinforces that schools of nursing need to convey the importance of quality clinical instruction for all faculty through mentoring programs and orientation sessions that are successful strategies to help new faculty socialize into their teaching roles. Fostering communication among all faculty and providing rewards for clinical teaching promotes the value of clinical expertise. Further studies are needed for faculty and clinical instructors to determine more effective teaching and learning methods for accelerated programs.

Rouse and Rooda (2010) examined factors for attrition in an accelerated baccalaureate program. These authors found that students in their 18-month full-time program had much higher attrition rates than the traditional program. The reasons as to why students did not graduate varied from personal or family health issues, academic dismissal, electing a part-time status, changing majors, and undisclosed personal reasons. The authors' recommended accelerated programs provide thorough orientation to students that emphasizes the program intensity and pace; first-hand testimonies from previous graduates; assistance with personal budgeting and financial resources; and counseling/stress reduction information and strategies.

METHODS FOR ASSESSING TEACHING EFFECTIVENESS

A systematic approach is needed to objectively assess the educational process. The educational objectives and their achievement outcomes are clearly identified with matching assessment techniques. Learners are provided with ample opportunities to meet the objectives and demonstrate outcomes. Multiple measurement techniques may be needed to assess some learning outcomes. The ultimate goal in assessing teaching/learning is to obtain valid and reliable information on the basis of which educational decisions can be made (McDonald, 2007). Assessment results can help direct and modify the teaching approach, the setting, and other amenable factors. Qualitative and quantitative data can be used. Efforts to evaluate teaching effectiveness have included student ratings; teacher self-evaluation; and student and graduate outcomes, such as examinations, certifications, employment, and other measures. The Center for Research on Teaching and Learning, University of Michigan http://www.crlt.umich.edu/tstrategies/tseot.php provides useful information about multiple methods for collecting data on teaching effectiveness.

Frameworks for assessing teaching effectiveness are lacking. Ogrinc and Batalden (2009) describe a realist evaluation as a framework for the assessment of teaching about the improvement of care to resident physicians and medical students. This framework from Pawson and Tilley provides an explanatory model that moves beyond a "yes" or "no," "does it work?" format to "what works, for whom, and in what circumstances?" that may identify the limits of when and where teaching interventions are effective. While this framework was used to determine if the educational program works and for whom, it has potential for further use in assessing faculty teaching effectiveness. Future studies are needed to determine how specific teaching strategies work best.

SELECTING AVAILABLE INSTRUMENTS

Student evaluations at the end of the course have been used as a measure of teaching effectiveness in most higher-education institutions for the last five decades (Smith, 2009). However, student evaluations are only a part of evaluating teaching effectiveness and may not be interpretable, as they often lack relevance, validity, and reliability. Major decisions, such as faculty placement in courses, promotion, tenure, awards, and merit increases, often rely on evaluations about teaching effectiveness (Smith, 2007). Careful design and testing of psychometric properties of such instruments provides educators with more confidence for their use. Emerson and Records (2007) provide a review of relevant teaching evaluation articles and the instruments used. Most of the instruments reviewed lacked adequate reliability and/or validity data. Smith (2007) studied end-of-course student ratings of teaching effectiveness and reported numerous similar problems. Emerson and Records' factor analysis of multiple classroom and clinical instruction evaluation forms explained "only 10% of the variance, leaving much unknown about teaching effectiveness" (p. 12). Both Emerson and Records (2007) and Smith (2007) reinforced the need to employ multiple methods of assessing teaching effectiveness using valid and reliable measures. These reviews illustrate the persistent need for better measurement instruments to assess teaching effectiveness.

Student biases have been reported as influencing their perceptions of teaching effectiveness. Sprinkle (2008) surveyed 202 students to determine how biases toward the educator's traits, for example, age, gender, teaching style, faculty ranking, personality, and grades affect their ratings of teaching effectiveness. Acknowledging limitations in small sample size, slightly skewed distribution, and other design limitations, this researcher found strong positive correlation between the awarding of "A" letter grades and traditional college-aged student ratings of teacher effectiveness. Sprinkle also found that as students' age increased, they were more likely to believe that educators over age 55 were more effective than younger students, who were more likely to believe that educators under 55 were more effective. As expected, if the educator's course information was disseminated in a manner congruent with the student's learning style, the student was more likely to rate the educator as effective. Educators who used humor, expressed concern and compassion, and showed interest in students both in and outside the course were rated higher than those not perceived demonstrating these personality characteristics.

Numerous paper-and-pencil types of instruments exist to measure teaching effectiveness. Bierer and Hull (2007) tested a clinical teaching effectiveness (CTE) instrument used for summative faculty assessment and found that the global item of the CTE correlated significantly with the factor scores. Therefore, these researchers "recommend reporting a global performance item if learners' ratings are used to make summative decisions about clinical teaching effectiveness" (p. 358). The reliability of another instrument measuring clinical teaching effectiveness (CTEI) developed to evaluate the quality of clinical teaching of educators in European medicine was found to achieve reliable findings and can be used to measure the quality of teaching (van der Hem-Stokroos, van der Vleuten, Daelmans, Haarman, & Scherpbier, 2005).

Berk (2005) critically reviewed 12 sources of evidence to measure teaching effectiveness: (1) student ratings, (2) peer ratings, (3) self-evaluation, (4) videos, (5) student interviews, (6) alumni ratings, (7) employer ratings, (8) administrator ratings, (9) teaching scholarship, (10) teaching awards, (11) learning outcome measures, and (12) teaching portfolios. He concluded that triangulation of multiple sources provided the best evidence. Faculty need to provide the most reliable base for making academic decisions and relying on only one or few sources should be employed with extreme caution. "Whatever combination of sources you choose to use, take the time and make the effort to design, execute, and report the results appropriately. The accuracy of faculty-evaluation decisions hinges on the integrity of the process and the reliability and validity of the evidence you collect" (Berk, 2005, p. 57).

Clinical competence of faculty has been identified as a measure of teaching effectiveness. Housel, Gandy, and Edmondson (2010) surveyed the importance of national credentialing in physical therapy students' assessment of clinical faculty effectiveness. These authors found that students rated the credentialed faculty significantly higher than the noncredentialed faculty. No similar studies for nurse faculty specific for credentialing were found.

Beran and Violato's (2009) study of 371,131 Canadian student ratings of teaching effectiveness, found that many factors determine how students rate their teachers. Using a well-established and tested Universal Student Ratings of Instruction (USRI) instrument, course characteristics such as length and type did not directly relate to student ratings. Student engagement, measured by student attendance and expected grade, did significantly relate to student ratings. When students were motivated and interested in a course, they participated more and had fewer absences. Students' engagement was higher in self-selected courses that required more work. The authors believed these courses involved more learning by the student about the subject.

A multidimensional approach to assess teaching effectiveness presents a better balance of important factors and thereby a more accurate view. Paper-and-pencil test (or computer administered), performance assessments, oral presentations, and portfolio assessment have been used (McDonald, 2007). Many teaching effectiveness instruments exist, few are psychometrically tested. Nurse educators are highly encouraged to use multiple methods in evaluating teaching effectiveness and to select instruments carefully with preference for well-established and tested instruments. It is critical to analyze the findings and use feedback to improve teaching (McKeachie, 2002). After implementing multiple methods in assessing teaching effectiveness, nurse educators are also encouraged to monitor for a pattern of teaching effectiveness over time, providing a more accurate representation.

ASSESSING THE OUTCOMES OF TEACHING EFFECTIVENESS

While all aspects of evaluation may be daunting, assessing the outcomes of teaching effectiveness poses one of the most important and challenging aspects of the faculty role. Teaching effectiveness is measured by the extent to which students have acquired specific learning outcomes (Bonnel, Gomez, Lobodzinski, & West, 2005). Faculty must provide fair and reasonable evaluation to determine student-learning outcomes. Nurse educators are charged with helping students prepare for current and evolving practice roles. Nurses must perform competently, appropriately interact with patients and various professionals, and adapt to ever-changing health care systems. Evaluation of outcomes needs to reflect these expectations. The quality of the student's performance is measured by assessing attainment of educational learning outcomes. Through evaluation, nursing educators can target additional educational needs to help students further develop competencies for practice.

Two forms of evaluation for students' learning may be made: formative and summative. Formative evaluation includes assessment of the student's progress during a course. This evaluation allows the nurse educator to identify competencies that have not been met, and develop a plan for enabling the student to achieve the required learning outcomes. Summative evaluation occurs at the end of the semester and provides the educator with an overall appraisal of competency level to base the final grade.

Assessment of outcomes should be the basis for completing a program. Educators enable students to achieve student outcomes. Most faculty members want well-educated graduates.

Eder (2004) reports his year-long search for identifying what university professors, corporate executives, and others believe graduates gain from their higher-education experience. Eder shared the following list of desired outcomes of high-quality university graduates compiled from professors and corporate people he has interviewed:

- Is a lifelong learner and has abiding curiosity;
- Possesses self-confidence and a sense of personal achievement;
- Exhibits and employs critical thinking;
- Is competent in written communication;
- Is competent in oral communication;
- Has a sense of ethics and responsibility;
- Knows something in some detail about a subject area (p. 136).

These graduate outcomes are desired by most educators, including nurse educators. Nursing educators value the competence and clinical reasoning ability of their students and graduates and view this ability as outcomes of their teaching effectiveness. Numerous models and strategies exist to increase clinical reasoning ability, critical thinking, and other similar concepts. Few have been tested. Bartlett et al. (2008) described an Outcome-Present State Test (OPT) Model of Clinical Reasoning designed to assist students in developing clinical reasoning skills. These authors tested the OPT in an undergraduate psychiatric and mental health clinical nursing course and found the model useful to students. Bartlett et al. recommend further research comparing the OPT model with other strategies that promote clinical reasoning.

Standardized patients (SPs) have also been incorporated in teaching as a method to increase student competence. Becker, Rose, Berg, Park, and Shatzer (2006) described a comparison of SPs with traditional paper-and-pencil measures of competence. In this pilot study, 147 senior undergraduate students in a psychiatric nursing course of a large mid-Atlantic university were randomly assigned to an SPs group or traditional group, and were pre- and posttested. No significant differences were found between the two groups on therapeutic communication skills, interpersonal skills, and knowledge of depression. However, students who participated in the SPs group overwhelmingly rated the experience as positive, creative, and meaningful. How students demonstrate competence and clinical reasoning varies widely. Observation, tests, simulations, and other methods are used. Karlowicz (2010) described the development and testing of a portfolio evaluation scoring tool for students to demonstrate their acquisition of nursing knowledge and skills in the nursing program. The psychometric properties of a self-evaluation of core competencies for baccalaureate nursing students was conducted by Hsu and Hsieh (2009) and reportedly could be used to assess core competencies of undergraduate nursing students.

FUTURE DIRECTIONS

The Institute of Medicine reports for nursing education (Finkelman & Kenner, 2007) provide important focus for accelerated programs. Preparing competent graduates for a continuously changing health care system poses challenges. Evidence-based teaching as described by Cannon and Boswell (2012), along with evidence-based practice, is our goal. Ferguson and Day (2005) present intriguing questions regarding evidence-based nursing education. Educators should be using the best evidence to assess their teaching and learning outcomes. Many challenges lie ahead as educators develop and implement best practices.

Integrating technology into future education and practice is essential (Mastrian, McGonigle, Mahan, & Bixler, 2011). Using online as a delivery method is gaining popularity. However, designing courses for online delivery requires effort and special considerations. Factors to consider (n.d.) in teaching online courses include:

- Motivation for the student: Why learn this? Where and when is this used? What are the payoffs for learning?
- Motivation for the faculty: What are the reasons for developing this course? How can you create the best learning experience for the students?
- Time: Preparing all materials ahead of time requires significant time commitment.
- Pedagogical considerations: What pedagogical models and learning theories are you incorporating into the teaching of the material?
- Orientation: Help the student adjust to the environment or content being taught, that is, preview, objectives, overviews, summaries, prerequisites, and schedule.

- Information: The content the student needs to master, that is, facts and evidence, demonstrations and skill steps, definitions and examples, evidence and cases, control and explain events, recall data, perform tasks, identify concepts, and infer outcomes.
- Application: How will the student demonstrate learning, that is, practice, prompting, feedback, remediation?
- Evaluation: How will you assess what the student has learned, whether the content was relevant, or whether the instructional method was appropriate?
- Technical competency: Are you comfortable with the technology used to deliver your course content? Will you need training or support?

Online delivery of courses is occurring at extraordinary speed. Educators are working diligently to measure its impact on learning. The impact of online delivery on learning outcomes is in its infancy stage with few well-designed studies available. One study comparing instructors' and students' perceptions of the effectiveness of online courses was conducted by Seok, Kinsell, DaCosta, and Tung (2010) and revealed that both had positive perceptions of course effectiveness. Flexibility, navigation, technical assistance, getting started, user interface, instructor and student course management, communications, universal and instructional design, and content were subscales of the instructors' and students' perceptions of course effectiveness.

Huckstadt and Hayes (2005) evaluated the effectiveness of two interactive online learning modules for 73 advanced practice nurses and found significant knowledge change scores from pretest to posttest. Learners evaluated the modules as innovative, time saving, convenient, available, and economical. Cook et al. (2008) used a meta-analysis of 201 eligible studies of Internet-based learning in the health professions and concluded Internet-based learning is associated with large positive effects compared to no intervention; however, when Internet-learning is compared to traditional methods, the effects are generally small. Currently, learning effectiveness is similar for Internet and traditional forms of learning. Further research is needed to determine how Internet-based learning can be effectively implemented and for what types of educators and learners.

McCurry and Martins (2010) described the successes of using innovative approaches to teaching undergraduate nurses in a research course compared to traditional approaches. Recognizing that the majority of current nursing undergraduate baccalaureate students are considered "millennial learners" born between 1980 and 2000, their view of the world is more global and multicultural. These millennial learners are considered more technologically adept and multitaskers who value doing rather than knowing. McCurry and Martins' innovative activities included collaborative learning, diverse clinical and professional clinical nurse researcher presentations, required participation with self-and-peer evaluations, joint assignments with corequisite clinical courses, oral group presentations and posters, research grand rounds, and an experiential learning assignment to introduce course topics for the semester. In comparison with traditional learning, students consistently rated the innovative approaches as more effective than the traditional one. Qualitative data revealed that students enjoyed and believed that the innovative activities were the most effective.

More sophisticated, realistic technology is valued by adult learners and will become more available in the future. Grady et al. (2008) examined teaching effectiveness as 52 first-semester nursing students were taught nursing nasogastric tube and indwelling urinary catheter insertion procedures using either high-fidelity (human-like physiological and vocal responsiveness) or low-fidelity mannequins (anatomical representations only). These researchers found that students had a higher performance with the high-fidelity mannequin and reported a more positive attitude. Accelerated nursing students value realistic hands-on experiences and would likely learn better using more sophisticated high-fidelity learning experiences. The closer the simulated learning experiences can mirror actual clinical situations, the better the learning experience.

Faculty toolkits similar to those described by Sager, Azzopardi, and Cross (2008) could be developed to foster teaching effectiveness in accelerated programs. Collaboration among the existing programs and those in development phases would benefit from shared resources. Learning and teaching resources that are targeted for diverse learners, teaching effectiveness instruments, and other related resources could be accessed. The challenge of how to help educators and students relate best in the education process will be met as we share what is known, what is available, and where we are heading in the future.

Online resources across the nation have become available. Educators are sharing resources for faculty and students at unprecedented speed and scope. The California State University Affordable Learning Solutions http://als.csuprojects.org/home is designed to enable the faculty to choose and provide quality educational content that is more affordable for their students. Faculty, staff, and students can access no/low-cost course content that can substitute for more costly learning materials. Another resource, Merlot (Multimedia Educational Resource for Learning and Online Teaching), http://www.merlot.org/merlot/index.htm, provides a wealth of peer-reviewed information for educators.

TABLE 4.1 Summary of Challenges, Strategies, and Future Directions for Achieving Excellence in Teaching

CHALLENGES	STRATEGIES	FUTURE DIRECTIONS
■ Rapidly evolving knowledge ■ Ever-changing healthcare environment ■ Novice faculty/clinical instructors transitioning to academia ■ Complex, multifactorial teaching–learning process ■ Difficulties measuring teaching effectiveness ■ Rapid increase in accelerated nursing programs and faculty shortage ■ Diverse learners ■ Evolving scholarship in nursing education ■ Outcomes of teaching effectiveness and academic decisions	■ Employ a wide variety of teaching/learning methods ■ Analyze feedback from variety of resources to improve teaching effectiveness ■ Consider diverse needs of learners and adjust teaching accordingly ■ Capitalize on learner's motivation ■ Evaluate teaching effectiveness through multiple sources and use valid and reliable instruments ■ Mentor novice educators to the academic role	■ Better evidence-based teaching and learning outcomes ■ Refined psychometric testing of measures to assess teaching effectiveness ■ Triangulation of multiple methods for assessing teaching effectiveness ■ Best practices for educators in accelerated nursing programs ■ Online resources in support of faculty development of teaching effectiveness ■ Lifelong learning for faculty to strive for teaching excellence ■ Institutional commitment and enhanced rewards for teaching excellence

The open educational resources are opening doors for students to take control of the learning process (Grush, 2011). Promoting "self-authorship" as a process of constructing the learner's own knowledge versus passively receiving knowledge should be the aim of education (Kolb & Kolb, 2005). Accelerated nursing students will be well positioned to take advantage of such resources. Teaching effectiveness will undoubtedly be affected by such resources. The challenge for all educators is to guide learners as they strive for increased learning experiences.

Table 4.1 summarizes challenges, strategies, and future directions for nurse educators striving to provide excellence in teaching.

REFERENCES

Bartlett, R., Bland, A., Rossen, E., Kautz, D., Benfield, S., & Carnevale, T. (2008). Evaluation of the outcome-present state test model as a way to teach clinical reasoning. *Journal of Nursing Education, 47*(8), 337–344.

Becker, K. L., Rose, L. E., Berg, J. B., Park, H., & Shatzer, J. H. (2006). The teaching effectiveness of standardized patients. *Journal of Nursing Education, 45*(4), 103-111.

Beran, T., & Violato, C. (2009). Student ratings of teaching effectiveness: Student engagement and course characteristics. *Canadian Journal of Higher Education, 39*(1), 1-13.

Berk, R. A. (2005). Survey of 12 strategies to measure teaching effectiveness. *International Journal of Teaching and Learning in Higher Education, 17*(1), 48-62.

Bierer, S. B., & Hull, A. L. (2007). Examination of a clinical teaching effectiveness instrument used for summative faculty assessment. *Evaluation & the Health Professions, 30*(4), 339-361.

Bonnel, W., Gomez, D. A., Lobodzinski, S., West, C., & Hartwell, D. (2005). Clinical performance evaluation. In D. M. Billings, & J. A. Halstead (Eds.), *Teaching in nursing: A guide for faculty* (2nd ed.) (pp. 521-542). St. Louis: Elsevier Saunders.

Bourke, M. P., & Ihrke, B. A. (2005). The evaluation process: An overview. In D. M. Billings, & J. A. Halstead (Eds.), *Teaching in nursing: A guide for faculty* (2nd ed.) (pp. 443-491). St. Louis: Elsevier Saunders.

Bradshaw, M. J., & Lowenstein, A. J. (2011). *Innovative teaching strategies in nursing and related health professions* (5th ed.). Sudbury, MA: Jones & Bartlett.

Cangelosi, P. R. (2007). Accelerated second-degree baccalaureate nursing programs: What is the significance of clinical instructors? *Journal of Nursing Education, 46*(9), 400-405.

Cangelosi, P. R., & Whitt, K. (2005). Accelerated nursing programs: What do we know? *Nursing Education Perspectives, 26*(2), 113-116.

Cannon, S., & Boswell, C. (2012). *Evidence-based teaching in nursing: A foundation for educators*. Sudbury, MA: Jones & Bartlett Learning.

Cook, D. A., Levinson, A. J., Garside, S., Dupras, D. M., Erwin, P. J., & Montori, V. M. (2008). Internet-based learning in the health professions: A meta-analysis. *Journal of the American Medical Association, 300*, 1181-1196.

Eder, D. J. (2004). General education assessment within the disciplines. *The Journal of General Education, 53*(2), 135-157.

Emerson, R. J., & Records, K. (2007). Design and testing of classroom and clinical teaching evaluation tools for nursing education. *International Journal of Nursing Education Scholarship, 4*(1), Article 12. Retrieved from http://www.bepress.com/ijnes/vol4/iss1/art12

Factors to consider. (n.d.). In *Virtual university design and technology,* University of Michigan, Teaching and Learning. Retrieved from http://vudat.msu.edu/teach/factors-consider

Ferguson, L., & Day, R. A. (2005). Evidence-based nursing education: Myth or reality? *Journal of Nursing Education, 44*(3), 107-115.

Finkelman, A., & Kenner, C. (2007). *Teaching IOM: Implications of the Institute of Medicine reports for nursing education.* Silver Spring, MD: American Nurses Association.

Forrest, S. (2004). Learning and teaching: The reciprocal link. *The Journal of Continuing Education in Nursing, 35*(2), 74-79.

Grady, J. L., Kehrer, R. G., Trusty, C. E., Entin, E. B., Entin, E. E., & Brunye, T. T. (2008). Learning nursing procedures: The influence of simulator fidelity and student gender on teaching effectiveness. *Journal of Nursing Education, 47*(9), 403-408.

Grush, M. (2011, March). Student-driven content. *Campus technology: Empowering the world of higher education. 24*(7), 50.

Hativa, N., Barak, R., & Simhi, E. (2001). Exemplary university teachers: Knowledge and beliefs regarding effective teaching dimensions and strategies. *The Journal of Higher Education, 72*(6), 699–729.

Housel, N., Gandy, J., & Edmondson, D. (2010). Clinical instructor credentialing and student assessment of clinical instructor effectiveness. *Journal of Physical Therapy Education, 24*(2), 26–34.

Hsu, L., & Hsieh, S. (2009). Testing of a measurement model for baccalaureate nursing students' self-evaluation of core competencies. *Journal of Advanced Nursing, 65*(11), 2454–2463. doi: 10.1111/j.1365-2648.2009.05124.x.

Huckstadt, A., & Hayes, K. (2005). Evaluation of interactive online courses for advanced practice nurses. *Journal of the American Academy of Nurse Practitioners, 17*(3), 85–89.

Karlowicz, K. A. (2010). Development and testing of a portfolio evaluation scoring tool. *Journal of Nursing Education, 49*(2), 78–86. doi: 10.3928/01484834-20090918-07.

Kolb, A. Y., & Kolb, D. A. (2005). Learning styles and learning spaces: Enhancing experiential learning in higher education. *Academy of Management Learning & Education, 4*(2), 193–212.

Kruszewski, A., Brough, E., & Killeen, M. B. (2009). Collaborative strategies for teaching evidence-based practice in accelerated second-degree programs. *Journal of Nursing Education, 48*(6), 340–342.

Lockwood, S., Walker, C. A., & Tilley, D. S. (2009). Faculty perceptions of an accelerated baccalaureate nursing program. *Journal of Nursing Education, 48*(7), 406–410.

Mastrian, K. G., McGonigle, D., Mahan, W. L., & Bixler, B. (2011). *Integrating technology in nursing education: Tools for the knowledge era.* Sudbury, MA: Jones & Barlett.

McCurry, M. K., & Martins, D. C. (2010). Teaching undergraduate nursing research: A comparison of traditional and innovative approaches for success with millennial learners. *Journal of Nursing Education, 49*(5), 276–279.

McDonald, M. E. (2007). *The nurse educator's guide to assessing learning outcomes* (2nd ed.). Sudbury, MA: Jones & Bartlett.

McKeachie, W. J. (2002). *McKeachie's teaching tips: Strategies, research, and theory for college and university teachers* (11th ed.). Boston: Houghton Mifflin.

Menix, K. D. (2007). Evaluation of learning and program effectiveness. *The Journal of Continuing Education in Nursing, 38*(5), 201–208.

Mullen, P. A. (2007). Use of self-regulating learning strategies by students in the second and third trimesters of an accelerated second-degree baccalaureate nursing program. *Journal of Nursing Education, 46*(9), 406–412.

Oermann, M. H., & Gaberson, K. B. (2009). *Evaluation and testing in nursing education* (3rd ed.). New York: Springer.

Ogrinc, G., & Batalden, P. (2009). Realist evaluation as a framework for the assessment of teaching about the improvement of care. *Journal of Nursing Education, 48*(12), 661–667.

Penprase, B., & Koczara, S. (2009). Understanding the experiences of accelerated second-degree nursing students and graduates: A review of the literature. *The Journal of Continuing Education in Nursing, 40*(2), 74–78.

Rico, J. S., Beal, J., & Davies, T. (2010). Promising practices for faculty in accelerated nursing programs. *Journal of Nursing Education, 49*(3), 150–155.

Roche, L. A., & Marsh, H. W. (2000). Multiple dimensions of university teacher self-concept. *Instructional Science, 28*, 439–468.

Rossetti, J., & Fox, P. G. (2009). Factors related to successful teaching by outstanding professors: An interpretive study. *Journal of Nursing Education, 48*(1), 11–16.

Rouse, S. M., & Rooda, L. A. (2010). Factors for attrition in an accelerated baccalaureate nursing program. *Journal of Nursing Education, 49*(6), 359–362.

Sager, S., Azzopardi, W., & Cross, H. (2008). Faculty toolkits. *Journal of Nursing Education, 47*(12), 576.

Schreier, A. M., Peery, A. I., & McLean, C. B. (2009). An integrative curriculum for accelerated nursing education programs. *Journal of Nursing Education, 48*(5), 282–285.

Seok, S., Kinsell, C., DaCosta, B., & Tung, C. K. (2010). Comparison of instructors' and students' perceptions of the effectiveness of online courses. *The Quarterly Review of Distance Education, 11*(1), 25–36.

Smith, B. P. (2007). Student ratings of teaching effectiveness: An analysis of end-of-course faculty evaluations. *College Student Journal, 41*(4), 788–800.

Smith, B. P. (2009). Student ratings of teaching effectiveness for faculty groups based on race and gender. *Education, 129*(4), 615–624.

Sprinkle, J. E. (2008). Student perceptions of effectiveness: An examination of the influence of student biases. *College Student Journal, 42*(2), 276–293.

Suplee, P. D., & Glasgow, M. E. (2008). Curriculum innovation in an accelerated BSN program: The ACE model. *International Journal of Nursing Education Scholarship, 5*(1), article 1, 1–13.

Tang, F., Chou, S., & Chiang, H. (2005). Students' perceptions of effective and ineffective clinical instructors. *Journal of Nursing Education, 44*(4), 187–192.

Van der Hem-Stokroos, H. H., van der Vleuten, C. P., Daelmans, H. E., Haarman, H. J., & Scherpbier, A. J. (2005). Reliability of the clinical teaching effectiveness instrument. *Medical Education, 39*, 904–910.

Vandeveer, M., & Norton, B. (2005). From teaching to learning: Theoretical foundations. In D. M. Billings, & J. A. Halstead (Eds.), *Teaching in nursing: A guide for faculty* (2nd ed.) (pp. 231–281). St. Louis: Elsevier Saunders.

Walker, J. T., Martin, T. M., Haynie, L., Norwood, A., White, J., & Grant, L. (2007). Preferences for teaching methods in a baccalaureate nursing program: How second-degree and traditional students differ. *Nursing Education Perspectives, 28*(5), 246–250.

Chapter
5

Recruitment, Retention, and Success in Accelerated Baccalaureate Nursing Programs

Kimberly J. Sharp and David M. M. Sharp

INTRODUCTION

*O*ver the past two decades, accelerated entry programs have proliferated throughout the United States (Lyon, Younger, Goodloe, & Ryland, 2010), but despite this the nursing profession is still unable to meet the demand for baccalaureate-prepared nurses (Siler, DeBasio, & Roberts, 2008). The push to introduce accelerated programs has been carried out in the absence of data on the efficacy and outcomes of these programs (Cangelosi & Whitt, 2005). This may be due in part to a lack of consensus on what constitutes an accelerated program (Schreier, 2009). Accelerated programs are designed for students who have previously graduated with a degree-level qualification. Penprase and Koczara (2009) note that accelerated programs are designed to capitalize on the students' prior experiences and learning and that there is some recognition of the students coming to the program as adult learners. Given the unique characteristics of this student population and the national demand for registered nurses, the means of attracting, retaining, and being successful with these students in accelerated programs gain increasing importance. This chapter will therefore examine issues that relate to the recruitment and retention of second-degree students and issues that influence their success as they move toward a new career in nursing.

Therefore, the following sections of this chapter will address topics of (a) recruitment to accelerated nursing programs, (b) retention within the programs and attrition issues, (c) disadvantaged students, (d) ensuring and measuring success, and (e) summary.

RECRUITMENT

Marketing Issues

Opportunities afforded in employment and salary and an accelerated route of nursing education are principle motivators for second-degree students choosing nursing as a new career (Lindsey, 2009). Having to invest their time, money, and effort to a second cycle of study, students are attracted to successful programs. Therefore, having sound programmatic outcomes along with a solid foundation for accelerated programs assists in the recruitment of new student populations. Any creative ideas for developing accelerated programs to generate income from new student pools cannot be implemented in a reactive manner. It is essential, therefore, to ensure sustainable growth opportunities for these programs and not merely the initial "flash in the pan" notes of interest prompted by something new. Cangelosi and Whitt (2005) outline the major problems associated with accelerated programs as being: competition for clinical sites, increased faculty workloads, program marketing, and inadequate screening of potential students. Therefore, any new accelerated program has to face the problem of being the "new kid on the block," as it attempts to promote credibility and access a portion of often sparse clinical opportunities. Faculty in existing programs may feel reluctant to become involved in the accelerated program if it is perceived that it may add to their already busy workload. This may be addressed by the institution recruiting additional faculty, but this may be problematic during the implementation of an accelerated program when the predicted revenues from the program have not yet been realized.

Accelerated programs attempt to attract candidates with degree-level qualifications. Recently, these may be people who have been affected by the downturn in the economy. The challenge for an educational institution is to reach out to these people who are contemplating nursing as a new, second, career choice and offer it as a viable option. Potential students may not even have contemplated nursing, or may not be aware of the possibility to study for a second undergraduate degree. Marketing should initially focus upon raising awareness of nursing as a second career, and outline how to enroll in and progress through an accelerated program.

Although marketing may generate initial interest in an accelerated program, that does not mean that all who become interested are suitable candidates. Some potential candidates may have an idealized notion of what the role of the nurse entails without ever having been aware of the job that nurses actually do. Having an introduction to nursing course as a prerequisite prior to entering an accelerated program offers potential nursing students the opportunity to gain insight into the role and skills expected of student nurses.

Candidates for the accelerated program, as with students applying for a place in a traditional program, may be initially accepted into the program but discontinued later if issues pertaining to health screening or a criminal background check are identified. For others, although they may have obtained a previous degree, they may be unfit academically or unprepared for the rigors and different study demands of a nursing program. This aspect of retention will be addressed later in the chapter.

Rosenberg, Perraud, and Willis (2007) stress that, with ongoing nursing and faculty shortages, "it is incumbent on colleges of nursing to make the best possible admission decisions—those that result in the highest possible retention rates of students well suited to the profession" (p. 413). They also stress that inadequate screening of potential applicants is high on the list of problems that accelerated programs face. Therefore, having followed through on curricular planning and approvals, it is imperative to set up pre-licensure student applicant protocols. These protocols need to clearly delineate what students must have in order to be eligible to apply for admission.

Recruitment to accelerated programs initially targets the local population to meet a perceived local demand. If a student lives locally, then that student is more likely to find out about the program. Realizing it can be accessed close to home also enables the student to make best use of their support system. Recruitment strategies can also be sensitive to changes in the local economy and can target specific sectors; for example, if a large production facility closes down locally.

A potential problem for accelerated programs is in recruiting from diverse and underprivileged sections of the community, especially during a national economic downturn. Potential students who have perhaps sacrificed and struggled to obtain a first degree, and have now established a level of economic security, may have fears about embarking on a second-degree program. There may not be opportunities for the support they require to complete a second degree and enable them to move from a closed, or limited, career path into a career in nursing with potential financial security. The financial challenges for accelerated students will be discussed in some detail later in this chapter, but it is necessary to note here that in terms of recruitment, many potential candidates for accelerated programs are reluctant to commit to such courses because of the potential financial hardships that need to be overcome. These candidates may still be in debt from their first-degree program, or have ongoing financial commitments and no access to scholarships, loans, or grants. This makes recruitment from diverse areas of the population a challenge for accelerated programs.

Increasingly, these programs are also attempting to recruit nationally through advertising their programs online and via the use of the Centralized Application Service for Nursing Programs, and being promoted by the American Association of Colleges of Nursing.

Admission Protocols

Admission protocols to accelerated programs normally include the following:

- Undergraduate degree specifications from an accredited college/ university and the discipline studied.
- Undergraduate degree parameters related to core curriculum, since some international programs do not require liberal arts exposure. This is an issue for accelerated programs that assume a broad educational foundation to have been acquired in the first undergraduate degree. For example, a student with a 5- or 6-year singular focus in ophthalmology may not have had that general education background knowledge.
- Currency of degree, if that is a factor for the college/university.
- Currency of prerequisite coursework obtained, either within or outside the degree earned. Some institutions make the decision to accept prerequisite coursework earned within the degree period, but for ad hoc prerequisites that are taken to meet entry requirements, those courses are to be taken within the last 5 years prior to commencing the program.
- GPA requirements, either cumulative or the last 60 hours. One tends to find that the last 60 hours can be a better measure of current functioning and reflect performance abilities on selected prerequisite coursework (usually sciences).
- Language proficiencies, such as TOFEL scores. Since some students through residency permissions may not be required to complete TOFEL assessments, interview profiling and other screening measures are recommended.

- Math proficiency assessment in basic competencies as part of, or distinct from, other entry assessment measures.
- Critical thinking performance assessment such as the Test of Essential Academic Skills (TEAS), the A2 HESI profile, or the California Critical Thinking Test. Each affords unique data that are illustrative to the institution, and helps to inform students of areas of weakness and those in need of remediation.
- Entry benchmark to compare with outcome data, using tools such as a combined Evolve Admission and Critical Thinking Test.
- A written goals statement is a useful tool in evaluating whether nursing truly is a good fit for the student. It is recommended that this be hand written when the student comes for an interview, as it ensures that it is an authentic piece of their own work, helps to assess illustrative writing and language ability, and gives the student an opportunity to share what motivates him/her to transition into the profession of nursing.
- Selection interviews can be conducted with individuals or groups. Group interviews can be more expeditious in terms of time management.
- Recruitment data should include demographic details regarding employment/career area prior to application. This will over time yield information for those recruitment areas with the greatest potential for students. So information sessions and marketing can become more targeted.
- Invitations to recruitment seminars can be promoted by offering special deals related to waiving or reducing application fees, and so on.
- A point weighting system for accelerated student applicants can be developed in order to streamline the application process on the basis of student ranking. This gives each student a ranked score in the profiling of all application data points and ensures greater transparency in the decision-making process related to student selection.

Admission criteria should be made available through the college/university website links, and other dissemination measures.

Publicizing Accelerated Programs

Publicizing accelerated programs may be through online sources, published materials, word of mouth, social media, and websites. A dedicated recruitment specialist or liaison person needs to be allocated to work with the accelerated students. To support the work of the accelerated recruitment specialist, information sessions for recruitment need to be promoted, and tri-monthly and special application meetings with individuals seeking clarification regarding transfer credits for transcripts should be conducted. Telephone message "voice blast" technologies related to upcoming workshops and/or promotions, or e-mail distribution lists can be sent out to candidates who have submitted contact details. The authors have experienced starting up an accelerated entry-level program in the northwest and central southern United States. Despite considerable interest in the initial start-up, few applicants were able to satisfy prerequisite requirements in time for the projected program start-up date, so a rolling program of applicants with projected application dates was put in place. After students have completed the full application packet with the elements outlined on the criteria sheet and supplied the required fees, a list of suitable prospective student applications for interview can be generated.

Recruitment to accelerated programs presents challenges in relation to raising awareness of the program, identifying suitable candidates for the program, completion of prerequisite courses by candidates, and providing the appropriate learning infrastructure in terms of faculty and learning opportunities. Potential students may be attracted to accelerated nursing programs for altruistic motives as well as the perceived potential financial rewards and job security within nursing. However, potential students must be apprised of the fact that entry to a nursing program is conditional upon satisfying mandatory health and criminal background checks and that the process of completing an accelerated nursing degree is challenging and different from their first-degree experience. There may also be financial challenges that have to be met during the course of the program, and these may be problematic when attempting to recruit potential students from minority and underrepresented sections of the population.

Having expended the time, energy, and planning on recruiting a cohort of accelerated nursing students, the institution must then ensure the continued viability of the cohort, and the program, as well as the eventual success of the students, by ensuring that the students are retained within the program.

Considerations in Interviewing

Interviewing potential students before admission may help identify those candidates best suited for an accelerated program (Penprase & Koczara, 2009). A range of noncognitive factors have to be considered and identified in the applicants (Jeffreys, 2002), including ascertaining if the candidate understands the commitment one is making and the life changes one may face, personal characteristics that help success in clinical practicum such as compassion, integrity, altruism, motivation, interpersonal skills, and respect. The interview process needs to be fair and free of bias (Rosenberg et al., 2007). A guided interview template is helpful to ensure consistency between the individual or group interviews. During the interview process candidates must be made aware of benchmarks for what the institution will accept as viable cohort numbers. Faculty workload and other resource decisions are derived from the projected tuition revenues and these must be commensurate with the projected needs in new program offerings. An added burden on faculty, such as changing course delivery methods within accelerated programs, often forces "nurse educators to adapt and learn at almost the same pace as the students they are teaching" (Rosenberg et al., 2007, p. 406). This factor needs to be considered when planning accelerated programs, and uncertain faculty add another level of stress on the students.

Cohort Viability

Students need to be apprised if the required numbers to commence an intake have not been met, and timelines for revised start-up dates need to be provided. Students expect the institution to provide accurate details about a program start-up. Accelerated students also need to be facilitated for their role transition from other career pathways and have enough lead time to make changes in their employment and/or family commitments. The anticipated number of accelerated students will need to be provided to admission and registrar offices so that they can work to have support systems in place for the incoming students. New courses or course numbers need to be built into the registration systems, and caps for student registration must be set. Ongoing updates and review data on the viability of candidate numbers necessitates clear communication across institutional divisions. There is always a level of fluidity between the student numbers required to meet program costs, the numbers anticipated by the registration documentation for application to the program, and the reality of the final totals of the "rear ends on seats," when students actually turn up for the first day of class.

The application data seek to affirm to all parties that accelerated candidates have the necessary abilities (intellectual, emotional, social, and physical), dexterity, and fortitude to complete the accelerated nursing program. Students requiring special accommodations through the declaration of documented disabilities will be required to achieve the same programmatic outcomes but will do so with the benefit of specific accommodations.

Motivation to Enter Nursing

Candidates are often attracted to entering an accelerated nursing program because of their desire to: "help people" or to have "patient contact" (Cangelosi & Whitt, 2005, p. 113); "find greater meaning in their work" (Miklancie & David, 2005, p. 291); "make a difference" and "have value" as well as "meaning" in their work (Aktan et al., 2009). Hammer and Bentley (2007) observe that in general the motivation of these students is based not only on economic reasons, but also an altruistic interest in entering a helping profession. Having this altruistic motivation for entering the accelerated program makes an even more compelling case for doing whatever one can to assist with student retention.

RETENTION

Retaining accelerated students requires consideration of the following:

Demographics

Accelerated nursing students address a particular demographic for considering student retention. American Association of Colleges of Nursing (AACN, 2009) states that accelerated nursing programs need to build on the content of previous undergraduate programs as well as learning experiences in order to provide an effective transition into a nursing program. Being an older group, with developed life experiences and personal commitments, more diverse, accelerated nursing students offer a unique set of challenges when it comes to retention in the nursing program (Cangelosi & Whitt, 2005; Siler et al., 2008). The majority of students are fairly recent graduates and bring successful previous knowledge and study skills into the nursing program. However, some students need to readjust away from previous study habits to learn and apply information in a different way in nursing education (Lyon et al., 2010). For example, for students with a science background, they have to think and write more like a student from the social sciences. Conversely, a student from humanities or social sciences may have to learn to think in a more scientific fashion, especially in relation to the science-based subjects such as anatomy and physiology that underpin a nursing program. Being out of school for a long time is considered a disadvantage, as students need to relearn study habits and readjust lifestyle to cope with becoming a novice learner in nursing.

Student Stress

Accelerated nursing students report more stress than students in traditional programs (Hegge & Larson, 2008; Masters, 2009). Sources of stress, apart from entering a new study area (Seldomridge and DiBartolo, 2007), may include the financial strain, a lack of available financial aid, and the expense of undertaking a second-degree program, especially if a student has to relocate from a region where he/she is settled (Lindsey, 2009). Stress is also caused by readjusting to the student lifestyle again, becoming novice learners in nursing, and struggling to pay student loans that are ongoing. These problems may be ameliorated somewhat if a student proceeds directly to an accelerated nursing program from a non-nursing program (Lyon et al., 2010). However, the relative youth and inexperience of the world outside academia might be a source of stress for these younger, direct-entry students. The only relevant experience they may bring to the nursing program is that of having been a student. Although this may have equipped them with a range of study skills, a support system, and the ability to survive financially as a student, they have not yet experienced the range of life experiences that occur after graduation when a person assumes a working role in society. They have not had to develop an alternative life outside the confines of academia and forge the relationships required to survive in the work arena.

The first clinical experiences for any student are highly stressful, but are especially challenging for adult students who have changed careers (Starr & Conley, 2006). Accelerated students have to acclimatize to clinical situations in a shorter time frame than traditional students and deal with the reality of changing careers while seeking to achieve at the high expectations that they have set for themselves (Caldwell, Tenofsky, & Nugent, 2010).

Stress management strategies have been beneficial for this group of students (Bradshaw & Nugent, 1997), with approaches such as reflection and introspection being used at the end of a class, and narrative approaches such as poetry, story, and song being used within the learning. The institution needs to understand stressors experienced by accelerated students, identify their preferred learning strategies, and assist faculty in facilitating the learning of these students (Weitzel & McCahon, 2008).

Transitioning into Nursing

Accelerated students have high expectations for themselves and may challenge "the critical thinking of faculty," forcing the faculty "to stay current in their teaching practices" (Bradshaw & Nugent, 1997). Shane (1983) put forward a returning-to-school syndrome model that helps in predicting the adaptation of accelerated students as they go through the developmental processes in this transition of returning to school and entering the field of nursing. In applying this model Utley-Smith, Philips, and Turner (2007) showed that in an accelerated nursing program there are three stages of development for the student, namely honeymoon, conflict, and reintegration. Knowledge of this process can assist nurse educators in predicting the path to be followed by accelerated students and help move them toward successful transition to the nursing program. Accelerated students may be more engaged in the classroom and may present a greater range of challenges for nursing faculty than those of non-accelerated students (Lindsey, 2009). Transparency in all of the recruitment information helps to ensure that programmatic expectations and the rigor of nursing course/clinical work are fully understood by students prior to their accepting an offer for admission. This is fundamental to student retention. Accelerated students may expect the educational process to be similar to their first degree (Lockwood, Walker, & Tilley, 2009). The student handbook is developed specifically to outline the expectations associated with the second degree.

Attrition Issues

Overall attrition rates are higher among accelerated degree students in comparison with traditional students (Suplee & Glasgow, 2008). Lindsey (2009) states that "attrition from accelerated programs typically is due to the rapid pace and intensity of the program, the program not being what the students expected, or students having unexpected personal issues" (p. 280). When accelerated student groups are taught as a distinct cohort, they develop their own culture and support network. However, when accelerated students are integrated into traditional preregistration student classes it is imperative that additional time is accorded to work with these students prior to integration. This process helps to address accelerated student anxieties and ensures that these students are properly orientated to nursing, along with the specific faculty and departmental expectations that sometimes can be more implicit than explicit.

Rosenber et al. (2007) argue that although attrition still occurs in accelerated BSN programs, these student outcomes could have been predicted from their applications or from the interview information. For example, a student who has excellent academic qualifications might never mention the caring aspect of nursing during the interview process and later fail a clinical practicum that eventually leads to exiting the program. Therefore, it would appear that awareness of the caring aspect of nursing is something that should be considered when interviewing potential students.

Understanding accelerated students helps reduce attrition rates. These adult learners grasp the relationships between concepts and courses and do not need the repetition that tends to be characteristic of traditional students, and they also appreciate being treated as adults in a collegial manner (Rico et al., 2010). They are experienced learners and therefore, in comparison, appear to be more verbal and assertive. Accelerated students seem to know what they want and what is expected of them. These students are mature and have to balance the demands of study, clinical, and home responsibilities that can include single-parent responsibilities or caregiver roles for elderly family members. They expect to have detailed schedules and time equivalency spreadsheets for each semester of study so that they can plan ahead for this array of responsibilities. They need clear guidance on study time expectations, and what the workload expectations are related to course and clinical assignments (Lockwood et al., 2009).

One of the major problems faced in orienting accelerated students to their program is when they note that we need to help "prospective students understand that such programs are accelerated, not abbreviated ..." (Meyer, Hoover, & Maposa, 2006, p. 327). These students must come to terms that they are undertaking a full program of study but the time available to do so is curtailed. Whenever course delivery templates for course sequencing and timelines need to be redeveloped in collaboration with available nursing faculty, then the draft schedules should be shared with the accelerated students so that they can plan for how the proposed changes may impact their domestic and other routines. Providing forums for student discussion about programmatic elements and ensuring that all students feel that their input is valued is a key aspect of student engagement in learning and in retention. The first month of adjustment into nursing study routines and introducing the accelerated students to the clinical environment can produce a high level of anxiety.

Accelerated students can have special challenges obtaining funding for study, since they may have exhausted grant/loan assistance for their first undergraduate degree. Indeed, finances and concerns related to financial support have played the largest role in accelerated student retention. Jeffreys (2002) noted that working full or part time provides added stress for students and affects retention. Seldomridge and DiBartolo (2005) reported that the average attrition rate for accelerated students was 10%. This is not a particularly high attrition rate, but what was surprising was a 25% no-show rate for fully accepted, registered, accelerated students not turning up on the first day of the program, a figure six times the rate for traditional students showing up for their program.

Accelerated students tend to be highly motivated but they do require continual feedback on how well they are doing in meeting targets. Prompt feedback, ongoing reassurance, and a positive approach with each student are key aspects of ensuring that they feel connected and supported. Retention is predicated upon the relationships built with students. Rouse and Rooda (2010) outline a range of interventions to decrease attrition rates in accelerated students, including a thorough orientation to the pace and intensity of the program; firsthand testimony from graduates of the program; one-to-one faculty mentoring; assistance with personal budgeting; and opportunities for counselling and stress relief. In addition, working with a nursing faculty advisor will help them to establish relationships that will make them feel more connected to the institution. Understanding students and always seeking to help them move toward their nursing goal sometimes means that they need to take time out for family, health, or monetary reasons.

Of course, the pace and intensity of a course are also major reasons for students to leave the course and the program. Be that as it may, Rosenberg et al. (2007) state that for accelerated students the "higher-than-desired attrition rates continue for a variety of reasons, for example, pace of program, poor lifestyle choices, and role concerns" (p. 413). Therefore, there are other than purely academic reasons that students cite for discontinuing an accelerated program, which include the need to work and earn some money, long commute times associated with attending the program, ongoing child and family responsibilities, and struggling with English as a second language (Rouse & Rooda, 2010). Attrition rates for these accelerated-degree students does require more research so that nurse educators can appropriately address and resolve the issues at hand as much for them as for the program.

Disadvantaged Students

Cangelosi and Whitt (2005) observe a distinct reversal in income levels after enrolling in an accelerated program. About 23% of participants in these programs had an income level below $16,000 before they enrolled. The low-income level jumped to 56% after students enrolled in the program. One of the biggest barriers to students accessing accelerated programs for a second degree is the lack of funding availability. Cangelosi and Whitt (2005) highlight a fact that all too many potential applicants for accelerated programs discover, that "graduate students are not eligible for many of the grant and scholarship opportunities of first-time college students" (p. 115).

Sources such as the Robert Wood Johnson Foundation promote new careers in nursing by targeting support for students in accelerated nursing programs. However, this funding is only available to students in programs with established NCLEX exam success, thus excluding newly established programs. In the authors' experience when establishing a new accelerated program, three disadvantaged students per year in the first two years of the program had to drop out because they had no source of funding to maintain them in the program.

Financial aid, especially in relation to the processing of loans/grants for students, causes other problems, as the authors' experience attests. When delays occur, and student loans/grants are not processed in a timely manner, for any number of reasons, it intensifies the stress that students must endure in this regard. It thus becomes critically important to ensure that the business office is appraised of any reason for payment delays. If the business office continues to send out invoices for the units of study that the students are enrolled in but do not yet have the resources in hand to pay for, this also can add to student frustration as they wait for the processing of funds.

Raines (2009) found that scheduling 12-hour clinical shifts on consecutive days produced demanding clinical practice hours that were a source of stress when combined with the demands of classroom-based courses and family needs. Economically disadvantaged students also face the further challenge of trying to find paid work that they can fit around the demands of weekly clinical commitments and the demands of continual study.

ENSURING SUCCESS

Ensuring student success involves academic progression and adequately preparing students to enter the nursing profession. "Maintaining the quality of an educational program, while decreasing the length of time for completion, is a delicate balance and likely to be closely scrutinized by the nursing community" (Cangelosi & Whitt, 2005, p. 340). Adherence to, and meeting, recognized standards is essential for sustaining the program. Some doubts exist among constituents regarding the success of accelerated programs in being able to produce successful students given the compressed nature of the program (Schreier, 2009). However, in support of academic institutions providing accelerated programs, Cangelosi and Whitt (2005) note that students in accelerated programs perform well, as supported by their high rates of passing NCLEX

(Bentley, 2006; Seldomridge & DiBartolo, 2005). The success of accelerated students in nursing programs is also related to high admission criteria, an entry GPA score of greater or equal to 3.5 on a 4-point scale (Mullen, 2007). These students have been successful in a previous program and continue with that level of success in the second-degree nursing program.

Students from other cultures undertaking an accelerated program may need special consideration, especially if their first language is not English. A climate of inclusiveness fosters self-affirmation and a sense of belonging for these students (Napierkowski & Pacquiao, 2010).

Bradshaw and Nugent (1997) highlighted a difference in learning needs for accelerated students in that they valued opportunities to expand patient teaching skills whereas traditional nursing students expressed a greater interest in acquiring technical skills. The traditional students were focused on learning how to perform the tasks of everyday nursing but the second-degree students were more interested in broader aspects of the nursing role. What was important in developing meaningful learning for accelerated students was to eliminate busywork associated with the nursing program (Lindsey, 2009). Some nursing schools need to tailor the curricula to meet the needs of accelerated students (McNeish, 2008). Lockwood et al. (2009) suggested that a Reflective Practice Model, as previously employed by Hobbs (2007), be used to address the unique learning needs of accelerated students. Suplee and Glasgow (2008) describe an innovative curriculum design for an accelerated program that heavily emphasized technology, professional socialization, and the use of standardized patient experience as a form of summative evaluation. They reported that over several years this 11-month program had considerable success with NCLEX pass rates.

Communication to students before, during, and after the program of study is the lifeblood to ensure their success. Students need to feel that faculty are eager for their success in the program, and that success and failure does matter, not just for them but also for the faculty. Outcomes cannot be compromised, but rejoicing in each milestone attained and sharing the successes of the accelerated cohort is crucial. Institutions may have wonderful resources but there also needs to be engagement between faculty and students, especially when dealing with mature students who have previously experienced a degree program. Students need to feel that they are the primary focus or they will walk. Lockwood et al. (2009) comment, "the accelerated students were more demanding of one-to-one faculty time for evaluation of both written assignments and examinations" (p. 409).

The selection of faculty who will seek to work with students and have a heart for creating a learner-centered learning environment is vital to ensure the success of students. Mentoring faculty in how to model and support student engagement can yield fantastic benefits. When students are engaged, they are eager to learn, participate in the classroom and clinical setting, and may challenge the faculty. Lindsey (2009) reminds us that accelerated students "tend to be highly inquisitive and tend to challenge the norms or status quo teaching and learning. As nurse educators this can be uncomfortable but the potential payoff is enormous" (p. 281).

As noted earlier, accelerated students may have more personal and family obligations than traditional students and absences caused by family illness or emergencies have a significant impact when the program of study is accelerated (Lindsey, 2009). These students need to develop self-regulating strategies in relation to developing appropriate learning experiences and clinical reasoning skills (Kuiper, 2005). Therefore, the institution needs to be aware of the contributions made by a range of variables that contribute to student success, including learner assessment, learning styles, and instructional strategies (Mullen, 2007), and plan accordingly.

The need for appropriate approaches to learning for accelerated nursing students is emphasized by Walker, Tilley, Lockwood, and Walker (2008), who describe the incorporation of novel and innovative strategies into accelerated programming that included a reflective practice framework, constrained optimization, modification of the clinical rotation model, waste reduction through efficient use of faculty and resources, contextual learning through integrated clinical course work, four semester themes, and the use of student-centered pedagogies that valued the depth and breadth of students' prior experiences.

To facilitate the achievement of goals set for accelerated students, it is important to work with students at all levels of the program. Initially, these students are very fearful of the clinical setting and the performance of actual patient care needs much reassurance and support, despite the fact that they might be successful in the classroom (Caldwell et al., 2010). Weitzel and McCahon (2008) discovered that accelerated students report clinical experiences as the most important component of the program. When improvements are necessary or issues do arise relating to clinical practice, frank and open discussion of key factors will allow students to vent concerns in a constructive manner. The use of supported clinical skills, lab facilities, simulation, and other learning systems all help to decrease student anxiety and facilitate learning. When it is possible to address student concerns in an expeditious fashion, that is always preferable, but when there is no immediate solution, being candid about recording the concerns in order to address these in the future may be one's only recourse. The key element is creating a climate that welcomes constructive and open communication in relation to the learning experience.

Faculty need to deal with issues the students identify with the accelerated program as these arise to prevent a feeling of uncertainty and frustration by the students. Continual dialog with the student group is therefore essential in promoting the partnership between faculty and the student group. The authors have found that having student representation on course committees creates structured opportunities for students to have meaningful input in program development and to develop themselves professionally.

Buonocore (2009) carried out a phenomenological study on a small group of graduates from an accelerated nursing program and outlined the following eight themes that emerged:

1. A "whirlwind" is forecasted in advance (regarding program requirements) but surprisingly unimaginable when it happens.
2. There is an awakening to the harsh realities of nursing through personal encounters with patients.
3. There is a "deer in the headlights" experience as students transform from novice to expert.
4. Mentoring from instructors, professors, and staff is highly valued.
5. The journey to the finish line ranges from easy to difficult depending on their previous career.
6. Students expect continuous quality improvement in the program.
7. Class camaraderie and the development of friendships ease the stress.
8. Overall, graduates liked the program and believe that they are better prepared to enter the workforce than traditionally educated nurses.

These themes were borne out as being familiar to the authors after having worked with accelerated students over a number of years. Looking at the experiences of accelerated students, teaching strategies that work for traditional 4-year nursing programs may not be so effective for adult learners in an accelerated second-degree program (Oermann, 2004). Wink (2005) remarks that this requires the accelerated students to complete a heavy course load each semester to be able to finish during the time allocated. Students in these programs must quickly adapt to the academic rigor and fast-paced program of study. Therefore, these students need to immediately put into effect their previously learned strategies for learning and socialize quickly into complex health care systems (Mullen, 2007). Certain groups of students are predicted to be more successful on the accelerated program than others. Lyon et al. (2010) observed that accelerated students perceived differing levels of difficulty in early nursing classes, with health science and basic science majors having an easier transition into nursing courses than students with other undergraduate degrees (2010, p. 1). Lindsey (2009) notes that "research is needed that examines the effectiveness of innovative curriculum designs and teaching strategies used in accelerated programs" (p. 281). Therefore, curricula for accelerated programs need to be redesigned rather than repackaged. This redesign needs to take account of the maturity and experience of the accelerated students, their preference for student-centered approaches to learning, and a mature relationship with faculty and clinical instructors.

MEASURING SUCCESS

Having attracted and recruited good candidates to the accelerated nursing program, it is anticipated that they will be retained and be successful through the end of the program. Rosenberg et al. (2007) maintain that accelerated programs are more successful than traditional programs in retaining students with "an average attrition rate of 10% to 15%, whereas traditional BSN programs average 20% to 30%" (p. 415). Rosenberg et al. (2007) recorded a clear link between cognitive measures, such as GPA and standardized test scores, and academic success in BSN programs, including success in NCLEX-RN, and that a number of studies have evaluated accelerated second-degree programs with similar results. Research is needed to measure outcomes of second-degree nursing programs. Accelerated programs are designed and accredited to ensure compliance with standards such as American Association of Colleges of Nursing essentials and Institute of Medicine competencies.

Keeping accelerated student data separate from the other preregistration student data helps to map any potential differences in overall performance. Newschwander (1988) in early time observed that not only did second-degree nursing graduates feel more competent in their jobs after graduation than traditional nursing students, but they were also being rated higher by their employers. More recently, the AACN (2010) noted that employers tend to prefer to hire graduates of accelerated programs and that these new employees are more likely to move into managerial roles more quickly that graduates from traditional programs. This could be due to accelerated students having more confidence in their role when they initially enter the work force, or it could be due to the richness of academic and life experiences that they bring to their new role in nursing. Raines et al. (2007) found that after entering the workforce these graduates had a higher rate of retention than expected for newly recruited staff and a large percentage of them planned on remaining at the bedside. Bentley (2006) noted that accelerated nursing students seemed to function at a higher clinical level than did their traditional counterparts. Korvick, Wisener, Loftis, and Williamson (2008) pointed out that accelerated students outperform traditional nursing students on a range of measures of success.

Other studies, such as those by Aktan et al. (2009) have found very little difference in outcomes between accelerated and traditional groups of nursing students following graduation, and Masters (2009) found that accelerated and traditional students enter similar fields of nursing and follow similar career plans. However, Lindsey (2009) notes that a number of studies have found that students in accelerated programs maintain higher grade point averages than traditional students and score higher on standardized nursing achievement. In 1995, McDonald found the pass rate on NCLEX-RN for accelerated nursing students to be significantly higher than that in the case of traditional nursing students, and this remains the case as confirmed by Lindsey (2009). Caldwell et al. (2010) noted that percentile scores on National League for Nursing exams are 10 to 25 points higher for accelerated, second-degree cohorts than for traditional students.

Critical thinking skills in accelerated second-degree nursing students have been found by Cangelosi (2007) to be higher than that for traditional nursing students, enabling them to move through the nursing program at an accelerated rate. Success can also be determined by retention data. If programs are given the autonomy to be able to retain and rechannel less successful, "decelerated," students into other preregistration routes, then these students would be assisted toward the achievement of programmatic outcomes. This serves to enhance student perceptions of institutional commitment to them, and ultimately promote the retention and reputation of the program. Accelerated students require this kind of consideration since they are unlikely to be attracted to a second nonprofessional degree outcome. Accelerated second-degree nursing programs are rigorous and effective (Penprase & Koczara, 2009); however, measuring the overall success of accelerated nursing programs remains problematic. After an extensive review of the available literature, Aktan et al. (2009) concluded that "the evidence of the effectiveness of accelerated programs compared to traditional programs is inconclusive; that is, we cannot conclude that one is better than the other. However, we can conclude from the evidence to date that both programs produce graduate nurses who have acceptable grade point averages and satisfactory pass rates on NCLEX" (p. 3). They go on to say that it is reassuring that, despite the compressed period of study for the accelerated students, they seem to have achieved the same level of socialization into the profession, as demonstrated in their commitment to their work as nurses and their level of professionalism.

CONCLUSION

Students who enter an accelerated nursing program do so for a variety of reasons that may be altruistic, financial, or personal. They have previously successfully completed a program of degree studies and therefore bring with them a range of study skills and strategies for academic success. Nursing education, however, often provides a different and challenging learning situation than that previously experienced. The content of the program may be delivered in more depth and at a faster pace than was anticipated. These students respond well to student-centered approaches to learning, where they take the initiative in their learning experience through strategies such as reflective journaling, group work, and problem-focused learning. Although these students may initially be intimidated by the new learning environment in nursing, especially in clinical areas, they quickly deploy their learning skills to come to terms with the process of becoming a nurse.

Accelerated students are a vibrant population of learners who seek to move beyond the task-focused and test-orientated preoccupation associated with most traditional student learners. They truly benefit from student-centered and creative opportunities in the teaching and learning environment. The curricula for accelerated students should be specifically designed to address their unique position as a cohort of mature, experienced, and successful students. Unfortunately, it is often more expedient to streamline the accelerated students within other student cohorts and follow the easiest, existing, path of delivery instead of widening the learning potential for these students.

REFERENCES

AACN. (2009). *Fact sheet: Accelerated baccalaureate and master's degrees in nursing.* Retrieved November 21, 2010, from http://www.aacn.nche.edu/Media/FactSheets/AcceleratedProg.htm

AACN. (2010). *Accelerated programs: The fast track to careers in nursing.* Retrieved December 14th, 2010, from http://www.aacn.nche.edu/Publications/issues/Aug02.htm

Aktan, N. M., Bareford, C. G., Bliss, J. B., Connolly, K., DeYoung, S., Sullivan, K. L. et al. (2009). Comparison of outcomes in a traditional versus accelerated nursing curriculum. *International Journal of Nursing Education Scholarship, 6*(1), 1–11.

Bentley, R. (2006). Comparison of traditional and accelerated baccalaureate nursing graduates. *Nurse Educator, 31*(2), 79–83.

Bradshaw, M. J., & Nugent, K. (1997). Clinical learning experiences of non-traditional age nursing students. *Nurse Educator, News, Notes and Tips, 22*(6), 40–47.

Buonocore, A. M. (2009). The lived experience of non-nurse College graduates in an accelerated nursing education program. Doctoral dissertation, University of Connecticut, 2009.

Caldwell, L. M., Tenofsky, L. M., & Nugent, E. (2010). Academic and clinical immersion in accelerated nursing program to foster learning in the adult student. *Nursing Education Perspectives, 31*(5), 294–297.

Cangelosi, P. R. (2007). Accelerated second-degree baccalaureate nursing programs: What is the significance of clinical instructors? *Journal of Nursing Education, 46*(9), 400–405.

Cangelosi, P. R., & Whitt, K. J. (2005). Accelerated nursing programs: What do we know? *Nursing Education Perspectives, 26*(2), 113–116.

Hammer, J. B., & Bentley, R. (2007). Lessons learned from 12 years of teaching second-degree BSN students. *Nurse Educator, 32*, 126–129.

Hegge, M., & Larson, V. (2008). Stressors and coping strategies of students in accelerated baccalaureate nursing programs. *Nurse Educator, 33*(1), 26–30.

Hobbs, K. (2007). The power of reflective practice in second degree nursing education. *International Journal of Human Caring, 11*(1), 22–24.

Jeffreys, M. R. (2002). Students' perceptions of variables influencing retention: A pre-test and post-test approach. *Nurse Educator, 27*, 16–19.

Korvick, L. M., Wisener, L. K., Loftis, L. A., & Williamson, M. L. (2008). Comparing the academic performance of students in traditional and second-degree baccalaureate programs. *Journal of Nursing Education, 47*, 139–141.

Kuiper, R. A. (2005). Self-regulated learning during a clinical preceptorship: The reflections of senior baccalaureate nursing students. *Nursing Education Perspectives, 26*, 351–356.

Lindsey, P. (2009 May). Starting an accelerated baccalaureate nursing program: Challenges and opportunities for creative educational innovations. *Journal of Nursing Education, 48*(5), 279–281.

Lockwood, S., Walker, C. A., & Tilley, D. S. (2009). Faculty perceptions of an accelerated baccalaureate nursing program. *Journal of Nursing Education, 48*(7), 406–410.

Lyon, D., Younger, J., Goodloe, L., & Ryland, K. (2010). Nursing students' perceptions of how their prior educational foci and work experience affected their transition into an accelerated nursing program. *Southern Online Journal of Nursing Research 2010, 10*(1), Retrieved from www.cinhal.com/cgi-bin/refsvc?jid=1911&accno=2010669304

Masters, J. C. (2009). Job satisfaction, job stress, burnout, and intent to leave among accelerated and traditional baccalaureate in science in nursing programs. Unpublished doctoral dissertation, University of Louisville.

McDonald, W. K. (1995). Comparison of performance of students in an accelerated baccalaureate nursing program for college graduates and a traditional nursing program. *Journal of Nursing Education, 34*, 123–127.

McNeish, S. G. (2008). Formation in an accelerated nursing program: learning existential skills of nuring practice. Unpublished doctoral dissertation, University of California, San Francisco.

Meyer, G. A., Hoover, K. G., & Maposa, S. (2006). A profile of accelerated BSN graduates, 2004. *Journal of Nursing Education, 45*, 324–327.

Miklancie, M., & David, T. (2005). The second-degree accelerated program as an innovative educational strategy: New century, new chapter, and new challenge. *Nursing Education Perspectives, 26*(5), 291–293.

Mullen, P. A. (2007). Use of self-regulating learning strategies by students in the second and third trimesters of an accelerated second-degree baccalaureate nursing program. *Journal of Nursing Education, 46*(9), 406–412.

Napierkowski, D., & Pacquiao, D. F. (2010). Academic challenges for culturally diverse students: A case study in one accelerated baccalaureate nursing program. *UPNAAI Nursing Journal, 6*(1), 9–10.

Newschwander, G. E. (1988). The accelerated option for non-nursing graduates leading to the Bachelor of Science in nursing degree: An analysis of the graduates' preparation and performance. Unpublished doctoral dissertation, Marquette University, Milwaukee, Wisconsin.

Oermann, M. (2004). Reflections on undergraduate nursing education: A look to the future. *International Journal of Nursing Education Scholarship. 1*(1), Article 5, Retreived December 12, 2010, from: http://www.bepress.com/cgi/viewcontent.cgi?article=1011&context=ijnes

Penprase, B., & Koczara, S. (2009). Understanding the experiences of accelerated second-degree nursing students and graduates: A review of the literature. *Journal of Continuing Education in Nursing, 40*(2), 74–78.

Raines, D. A. (2009). Competence of second degree students after studying in a collaborative model of nursing practice education. *International Journal of Nursing Education Scholarship, 6*(1), 1–12.

Raines, D. A., Sipes, A., & Christine, E. (2007). One year later: reflections and work activities of accelerated second-degree Bachelor of Science in nursing graduates. *Journal of Professional Nursing, 23*(6), 329–334.

Rico, J. S., Beal, J., & Davis, T. (2010). Promising practices for faculty in accelerated nursing programs. *Journal of Nursing Education, 49*(3), 150–155.

Rosenberg, L. R., Perraud, S., & Willis, L. (2007). The value of admission interviews in selecting accelerated second-degree baccalaureate nursing students. *Journal of Nursing Education, 46*(9), 413–416.

Rouse, S. M., & Rooda, L. A. (2010). Factors in attrition in an accelerated baccalaureate nursing program. *Journal of Nursing Education, 49*(6), 359–362.

Schreier, A. M. (2009). An integrative curriculum for accelerated nursing education programs. *Journal of Nursing Education, 48*(5), 282–285.

Seldomridge, L. A., & DiBartolo, M. C. (2005). A profile of accelerated second bachelor's degree nursing students. *Nurse Educator, 30*(2), 65–68.

Seldomridge, L. A., & Dibartolo, M. C. (2007). The changing face of accelerated second bachelor's degree students. *Nurse Educator, 32*(6), 240–245.

Shane, D. L. (1983). *Returning to school: A guide for nurses.* Englewood Cliffs, NJ: Prentice-Hall.

Siler, B., DeBasio, N., & Roberts, K. (2008). Profile of non-nurse college graduates enrolled in accelerated baccalaureate curricula: Results of a national study. *Nursing Education Perspectives, 29*(6), 336–341.

Starr, K., & Conley, V. M. (2006). Becoming a registered nurse: The nurse extern experience. *Journal of Continuing Education in Nursing, 37*(2), 86–92.

Suplee, P. D., & Glasgow, M. E. (2008). Curriculum innovation in an accelerated BSN program: The ACE model. *International Journal of Nursing Scholarship, 5*(1), 1–13.

Utley-Smith, Q., Philips, D., & Turner, K. (2007). Avoiding socialization pitfalls in accelerated second-degree nursing education: The returning-to-school model. *Journal of Nursing Education, 46*(9), 423–426.

Walker, C., Tilley, D. S., Lockwood, S., & Walker, M. B. (2008). An innovative approach to accelerated baccalaureate education. *Nursing Education Perspectives, 29*(6), 347–352.

Weitzel, M. L., & McCahon, C. P. (2008). Stressors and supports for baccalaureate nursing students completing an accelerated program. *Journal of Professional Nursing, 24*(2), 85–89.

Wink, D. (2005). Accelerated nursing programs for non-nursing college graduates. In M. Oermann & Einrich (Eds.), *Annual review of nursing education* (Vol. 3, pp. 271–279). New York: Springer Publishing.

Chapter 6

The Faculty Experience: Thriving in the Midst of Intensity While Pursuing Excellence

Cheryl L. Brandt, Melissa R. Boellaard, and CeCelia R. Zorn

*D*eep into a clinical rotation on the ortho-surgical unit with eight students in the accelerated baccalaureate nursing program (ABSN), Claire began to close the day. As a seasoned classroom and clinical educator, she and the students cared for patients recovering from hip and knee replacements, aortic aneurysm repairs, and above-the-knee amputations. Claire elegantly shaped every moment to teach and learn. She dedicated the shift to drawing connections, reviewing skills, practicing priorities, and affirming students' personal and professional development. Throughout the day, both students and patients confronted the bony balance of frailty and vigor, the many faces of loss and recovery.

Now the clock nudged mid-afternoon. Long past a lunch break that did not happen, Claire slipped into the report room, hoping to pilfer a few minutes of respite. Here she found Allison, one of the students reporting off to the day shift RN.

Throughout the shift, Allison cared for a 62-year-old woman who had a complicated bowel surgery the previous day. In her report to the RN, Allison meticulously detailed her assessment of the patient's body systems and the interventions she carefully provided over the past seven hours. As part of her report-off, she described the plan for the next IV bag. Referring to the next liter that she placed on the patient's

IV pole, Allison simply stated, "I hung the next IV bag in her room, but I didn't tap it yet."

With pen hovering above scribbled notes, the RN lingered and raised a haughty eyebrow. She peered at Allison over her glasses with a bit of sneer and a hint of mock. "Boy, I bet you've done *that* many times before." The RN was referring to Allison's use of the term "tap," equating it to "tapping or opening a keg of beer." The term used on this unit was "spike," as in spiking a new IV bag. Perhaps the RN regarded the term "tap" as peculiar, even a shortcoming, but without a doubt, she stuffed it with a college-age drinking stereotype.

Allison gulped, gathering her composure in the awkward moment. "Well, in fact" she replied with poise and resolve, "I probably did tap a few beers when I was a young college student back in my first degree, but now I have a 6-year-old daughter and those first college days only faintly shadow in my long distance rear view mirror."

Claire jolted to attention. She had just bumped headfirst into a dreadful communication that often occurs when we hold unswerving stereotypes. Silently, but with strike and smack, Claire challenged herself with several questions: "This regrettable interaction exposed some unique characteristics about *students* in the ABSN program. But what does this mean for me as a nurse educator? What stereotypes might I hold? How can I better understand who the students are and help others understand them also? How am I teaching and learning with these students? Might there be more effective ways of teaching?"

The purpose in this chapter is to examine the following statement: Faculty excellence builds on truthful and courageous self-reflection, listens ardently to student voices, and intentionally crafts educational experiences to enhance student learning and support their transitions. To begin the discourse, three major sections will be discussed: (a) a brief literature review related to ABSN education, (b) three educational frameworks to serve as a theoretical basis, and (c) a collection of stories that describes our experiences as ABSN educators.

REVIEW OF LITERATURE

We searched the literature focusing on the faculty experience with teaching ABSN students. In collaboration with a reference librarian, we used combinations of various key words (e.g., accelerated nursing programs, accelerated nursing, nursing curriculum, faculty, second-degree program, second-degree nursing, perceptions) in several databases: CINAHL, MEDLINE, ERIC, Education Full Text, and Dissertation Abstracts.

We reviewed 28 articles from 1989 to the present. Nearly 90% ($N = 25$) of the articles were published in the last decade; as a matter of fact, the majority ($n = 20$; 71%) were published in the last five years (i.e., 2006–2010). This current literature surge parallels a recent rise in ABSN programs and reflects a generally half-and-half split between nonresearch-based articles and those reporting research conducted with ABSN students, graduates, and faculty. As we were interested in content about the faculty experience, we used the following domains to structure our literature review: (a) nursing disciplinary expertise, (b) course/curriculum design and development expertise, (c) instructional practices, and (d) learning/teaching environment.

Overall, the ABSN literature is descriptive in nature. The primary focus has been to describe (a) programs and (b) students. Several themes were noted in ABSN program characteristics and curricular issues. For example, program models included a direct-entry MSN program for second-degree students (Schreier, Peery, & McLean, 2009) and collaborative partnerships between higher-education and health care agencies (Murray, 2007; Raines, 2006). In addition, authors have emphasized key curricular components in ABSN programs: (a) critical thinking (DeSimone, 2006; Miklancie & Davis, 2005; Suliman, 2006); (b) condensing, but not "double-teaching," content (Hamner & Bentley, 2007; Lockwood, Walker, & Tilley, 2009); (c) integrating ABSN with traditional BSN students (Rodgers, Burson, & Kirschling, 2004; Walker, Tilley, Lockwood, & Walker, 2008), and (d) professional socialization (Suplee & Glasgow, 2008; Utley-Smith, Phillips, & Turner, 2007).

Finally, in the program-focused literature, staffing considerations were also addressed. Lockwood et al. (2009) described the use of faculty for teaching theory and adjunct faculty for teaching clinical. Two authors also discussed using hospital staff to assume clinical teaching responsibilities (Murray, 2007; Raines, 2006).

In addition to program descriptions, many authors have described ABSN student characteristics. For instance, Lindsey (2009) portrayed ABSN students as "older learners who are more engaged and challenging in the classroom" (p. 280). Other authors have also highlighted ABSN students as adult learners (Vinal & Whitman, 1994) who (a) value challenging and meaningful assignments (Cangelosi, 2007a, 2007b) and (b) experience the "Returning to School" Syndrome (Utley-Smith et al., 2007). Furthermore, more than traditional students, the ABSN students prefer classroom structure, faculty direction, case studies, learning from faculty stories, and "learning for learning's sake" (Walker et al., 2007, p. 249).

Although most of the student-focused literature highlighted their demographics, experiences, and preferences for teaching techniques, one study examined stressors and supports for ABSN students. Weitzel and McCahon (2008) surveyed and interviewed ABSN students ($N = 69$) to describe factors that students believed contributed to their stress and contributed to students' supports. In this study, students identified too many writing and reading assignments, heavy workload and family responsibilities, the fast paced and intense program, and group assignments. Student supports included individual faculty and peers, advisors, class lectures, and families.

The emerging body of literature deepens an understanding of ABSN nursing education, particularly about program features, selected curricular components, and student characteristics. Only one study was retrieved that was specifically designed to investigate the experience of ABSN faculty as described in their own words (Cangelosi & Moss, 2010). Using a hermeneutical phenomenological approach, these researchers interviewed 14 second-degree ABSN faculty. Two themes reflecting challenges associated with teaching ABSN students emerged: "at the top of my game" and "teaching to think like a nurse."

Much of the information about the faculty experience of teaching was included only incidentally in articles written for a purpose other than to describe that experience. For example, common beneficial faculty characteristics were highlighted: clinical expertise, self-confidence, flexibility, dedication, sensitivity to students, and ability to manage intense workloads. Further, several constructive faculty approaches were also noted. That is, faculty were effective when they (a) communicated clearly, directly, and in detail; (b) created varied and nonduplicative learning experiences that were relevant to practice; (c) gave students latitude and built on their pasts to prepare for their futures; and (d) supported students' transitions and stressors.

In reviewing the literature, then, we concluded that it is a recent mixture of research and nonresearch articles that is growing rapidly and focuses largely on students and program descriptions. Our discussion in this chapter extends this foundation by emphasizing the faculty experience.

THREE EDUCATIONAL THEORIES: A BRIEF SUMMARY

Three commonly used educational theories provide a context for our discussion. These include Knowles' Adult Learning Theory, Constructivism, and Humanism.

Groundbreaking work by Malcolm Knowles first identified adult learners as a population with distinct characteristics and needs unique from those of their younger counterparts (Knowles, Holton, & Swanson, 2005). Knowles maintained that adult learners innately utilize their lived experiences as foundations for incorporating new knowledge to solve real-life problems. Adult learners are described as self-directed, autonomous, free thinkers who desire to be actively engaged in planning and evaluating their learning. Their motivation to learn is more problem centered and immediate. It is directly correlated to perceived usefulness or relevance of the content to their problem; in other words, the greater the sense of utility, the stronger the desire to learn. Adult learners approach learning as a means of achieving a specific goal; often that goal is associated with social or occupational competencies.

Unlike adult learning theory, which emphasizes problem centeredness and usefulness as motivation for learning, constructivism views learning as a developmental process. Learners "construct" new knowledge by interpreting or making sense of an experience as it builds on what they already know (Vygotsky, 1962, 1978). Vygotsky described the zone of proximal development (ZPD), which indicates what the student *could* demonstrate, learn, or perform with someone else's assistance. The ZPD includes those abilities that are in the *process* of maturing. These capacities reveal "the 'buds' or 'flowers' of development rather than the 'fruits' of development" (1978, p. 86); that is, the ZPD estimates things likely and forthcoming.

There is one primary component of constructivism: learning and developing higher levels of thinking are supported by assisted performance—this is termed as "scaffolding." As a striking metaphor for teaching, a scaffold refers to the temporary framework of planks and lumber that braces up construction workers and their supplies as they build homes and repair existing structures. In education, then, teachers design scaffolds that help students perform tasks or think in ways that would not have been possible otherwise.

For example, Hydo, Marcyjanik, Zorn, and Hooper (2007) used art as a scaffold to help students think in a new way. Beginning baccalaureate nursing students ($N = 91$) were asked to use "any art form to create a personal expression of what nursing is for them" (p. 3). The researchers concluded that "art served as a catalyst for re-thinking self-imposed boundaries" (Hydo et al., 2007, p. 9). It is likely that the art, the prompting questions, and the one-week time span all served as scaffolds for students' learning. These scaffolds called forth students' thinking in more profound and insightful ways than if they were simply asked to verbally respond on-the-spot to the question, "What does nursing mean to you?"

Finally, in contrast to adult education theory and constructivism, humanism is both a philosophy of and approach to education. As a philosophy, humanism is a commitment by teachers to students. In this commitment teachers accept responsibility for students; in essence teachers are "being for the other" (Safstrom, 2003, p. 28). In other words, teachers, from a humanist perspective, are student centered (Vandeveer, 2009).

As an approach to education, humanistic teaching occurs within student–teacher relationships. Safstrom (2003) emphasized the importance of interaction and dialogue. In the context of relationship, teachers guide, help, supervise, and encourage students (Ediger, 2006). Teachers design learning experiences and model desired behaviors, thus creating an environment that motivates students to learn.

Humanistic education is consistent with the nursing profession's focus on caring (Watson, 2000). In fact, Kleiman (2007) contended that students who see humanism modeled by their nursing instructors are better prepared to give humanistic nursing care to their patients. In other words, as the teacher is "for" the student, the nurse is "for" the patient.

Nursing educators have proposed models to integrate humanistic educational philosophy and practice with nursing education. Clark (2005) offered a "partnership model" as an alternative to a hierarchical, authoritarian, "dominator model" of teaching. In Clark's model, students are co-learners with peers and faculty, engaging in problem solving and reflection. Kleiman (2007) proposed a Humanistic Teaching Model in which self-actualization is the goal for students. In Kleiman's model, teachers and students are in a respectful relationship; they learn together through engagement, dialog, and exchange. Teachers encourage reflection and classes are shared research adventures.

These three educational theories offer distinct views on teaching and learning. Adult learning theory underscores the student as a self-directed learner who is motivated to solve problems and considers relevance and utility as key. Constructivism highlights the "potential and possibilities" of learning; with scaffolds, or assistance from the teacher, the student thinks or performs in ways not otherwise possible. Teachers who embrace humanism as a philosophy and an educational approach commited to students hold the student–teacher relationship in highest regard, and view educators and students as co-learners.

IN OUR OWN WORDS: DISCLOSING STORIES AND CREATING CONNECTIONS

Theories are one thing; experiences are quite another. There is no greater reality check for us as educators than to be struck head-on by a true "a-ha moment." "A-ha moments" are those precious instances when the light bulb not only goes on but glows so brightly that it hurts to look at it directly for fear that we might not like what we see. Or, they are occasions when we feel like someone just opened our eyes to something that is so blatant that we cringe because we did not notice it sooner. Those moments rock our confidence in what we thought we knew and give us a huge dose of humility. "A-ha moments" happen continuously, in every context of our lives, and we are changed as a result. The stories that follow are our "a-ha moments" related from a first-person faculty perspective. Fictitious student names are used.

Melissa's Story: "It Will Be Nice to Feel Competent Again"

While teaching ABSN students over the past couple of years I have had my share of "a-ha moments," and because of them I changed how I teach, how I relate, and how I connect with students. These moments enlighten my perspective of what it means to be an educator in an ABSN program and remind me that I have just as much to learn from the students as they have to learn from me.

During an e-mail conversation, Brandon told me how difficult it was to absorb the plethora of information we had covered that week in class. Overwhelmed by the amount of new content presented, the prospect of beginning to apply that content in practice, and ultimately needing to demonstrate content mastery on an exam in just a few days, he made the following statement regarding his upcoming shifts working in a pathology lab, ". . . it will be nice to feel competent again."

As I sat reading his e-mail that Friday night, I had an "a-ha moment." Some students I deem as novice student nurses are actually experts in another field. Many of these "novices" not only struggle with mastering course requirements, but also face the challenges of identifying themselves as professionals in an entirely new field. Lockwood et al. (2009) stated that the differences between ABSN students' previous employment or academic experiences and the professional environment of the baccalaureate nurse further complicate this challenge. In addition to the usual stressors, students also experience the vulnerability, uncertainty, and angst that go along with being a novice again. Cangelosi and Moss described this observation in their research; ABSN students "are in the unique position of having been experts in their previous fields and are now novices in both a rigorous academic program and a new profession" (2010, p. 141).

Consistent with adult learning (Knowles et al., 2005), we must help adult learners by facilitating, not managing, their learning. We need to guide their learning journey while suppressing our urge to designate the path by which the learner gets there. I discovered that I am most effective as an educator of adult learners when I am not simply the supplier of the facts but the nurturer of the seed of discovery. It is my job to ask the right questions, not just supply the right answers. I am "at the top of my game" when I respect adult learners by acknowledging the abundance of experience they bring with them and enthusiastically identifying how our collaborative learning is enriched.

Cheryl's Story: Moving Beyond Defensiveness Toward Liberation

As Melissa has reflected on the role of nursing faculty with ABSN students, my story is more about the feelings ABSN faculty experience. I have learned that feeling defensive does not help a teacher of nursing teach "otherwise" (Safstrom, 2003). It is challenging to focus on creating student-centered learning experiences, a goal of humanistic education, when I am focused on how bad I am feeling.

I will explain. In an attempt to both turn a testing situation into a learning situation and to model continuous exam quality improvement, at CeCelia's suggestion I began holding in-class exam reviews with the ABSN students. I had never done this before. A number of factors, including larger class size and the two-site character of student cohorts, had mitigated against, at least in my mind, attempting such an exercise with our traditional BSN students. With the ABSN students I had a smaller cohort, all in the same room, and all were adults taking their education, including the exams that were part of it, very seriously.

To be honest, I did not ask the ABSN students whether they had ever been part of an in-class face-to-face exam review the first time we held a review. I do not know if they were feeling as anxious as I was. In a real sense my work (the exam that I had created) was being held up for public critique and comment. I did not stop to think, of course, that as a teacher almost all of my work is public and thus open for public critique and comment.

We reviewed the exam, item by item. The students called out the correct answers and then identified items for which the stem had been difficult to interpret or responses were unclear.

I recall having felt defensive during that first exam review. My level of tension rose, my voice got sharper as it was clear that students had issues with some of the items. I recall needing to "talk myself down" as we finished the review, to remind myself that the students were not attacking me, only offering the critique of the exam that I had invited. I ended the session by further inviting the students to send me an e-mail citing a textbook reference or a section in their class notes that supported their selection of item responses I had deemed incorrect. I was prepared to throw out items for which the students made a justifiable argument.

I have reflected often on that first exam review; it has taken on deep meaning for me. It has come to represent a commitment to collaborative learning, an example of a teacher abandoning an authoritarian "what I say goes" stance for a collaborative "I may be wrong; help me do better" stance (Clark, 2005). It was a deliberate attempt to humbly engage with the students in a respectful relationship, learning together through engagement, dialog, and exchange (Kleiman, 2007). These are core tenets of humanistic education theory; they reflect the teacher's commitment to teaching "otherwise"—to being "for" the student (Safstrom, 2003).

Ultimately, it was liberating to admit that my exam items might not all be good. I observed a level of respect for the process from the students that I think reflected their appreciation of my willingness to accept their help in improving the exam. Feeling liberated and respected puts me in a better place to be a teacher "for" the students.

Melissa's Story: Evaluation as a Double-Edged Sword

My experience teaching ABSN students has also been liberating. However, my liberation came on the blade of the double-edged sword of evaluation. (My apology for the war metaphor but it figuratively describes the emotions I experienced.) As in any nursing program, we expect evaluation to be comprehensive, equitable, and consistent. In a small student cohort the expectations for faculty inter-rater reliability and equality gain even greater prominence. Ensuring that evaluation methods maintain these standards weighs heavily upon my shoulders.

As a result, I have collaborated extensively with my colleagues to develop, test, revise, and evaluate the effectiveness of our evaluation tools. This is a painstaking process. Not only is it time consuming, but it is also labor intensive and often frustrating. However, the substantial investment is well worth the reward when I am able to defend an evaluation tool to a group of disgruntled students claiming that they were unfairly evaluated. Despite my best efforts, it is sometimes difficult to maintain my composure and remember that what I may deem as a "full onslaught attack" is not directed toward me personally. It is directed toward the perceived unfairness of the evaluation tool.

Students also experience this "attack phenomenon" but with a different twist. For example, Katie received a poor grade on a medication calculation quiz and confronted me, "I'm not wrong! My answer is mathematically correct!" even though her answer was not clinically practical. Unfortunately, we were at an impasse. Later that day Katie e-mailed me and insightfully described what caused her initial reaction. Although she acknowledged her calculation error, she wrote, "As soon as I saw two red marks on the page I became defensive and felt personally attacked."

At that moment I saw evaluation as a double-edged sword. For Katie the quiz represented an extension of herself and she was unable to suppress the urge for self-defense. As Katie felt attacked *with* an evaluation tool, I have often felt attacked *about* an evaluation tool. In both cases the tool represented us. I realized that distinct perceptions from both sides of the evaluation battlefield carry high stakes which are exaggerated in an intense academic program. This realization was liberating and helped me see that one little flick of the wrist can turn a seemingly unthreatening evaluation tool into a harmful weapon that wields the power for mass destruction.

This experience is an example of one of the defining characteristics of adult learners. According to Knowles et al. (2005), adult learners are actively engaged in planning and evaluating their learning. When they are involved in the process of evaluation they feel less threatened, more engaged, and ultimately have more successful outcomes. For me, I will bear my scars with honor as testimony to continual collaboration with students around evaluation and leave the animosity on the battlefield.

CeCelia's Story: The Beauty and the Beast of the Nursing Profession

Building a clinical experience does not stop with providing direct care for patients and families. Nowhere does this seem more striking than with ABSN students in their condensed program—where the clock rapidly ticks the hours away, months melt, and seasons shrink. I feel called to make every instant count, designing a "clinical experience" that happens everywhere students can practice to be leaders.

Socialization of ABSN students as leaders in the profession has been recognized, albeit meagerly. Admittedly, the need for preparing nurse leaders has been depicted. Lindsey (2009) declared that nursing education must change "to challenge second-degree students, who will comprise a good proportion of the nurse clinical and academic leaders of tomorrow" (p. 281).

At the same time, the compressed time frame has been named as a barrier—"one year is not enough time to socialize students into the nursing profession" (Miklancie & Davis, 2005, p. 293). Rodgers et al.

(2004) insightfully noted a second consideration: because ABSN students come to study nursing from another discipline or profession, we may question how that influences their view of nurses as leaders. Finally, acknowledging the need for socialization, others have described their efforts to (a) encourage ABSN students in School of Nursing activities, (b) integrate ABSN students in classes with traditional students, and (c) create concentrated clinical experiences (Hamner & Bentley, 2007).

Over the past two years, my colleagues and I have had several experiences designing "out-of-class" socialization activities to immerse students in a professional life. Our emphasis was to literally transport them off the campus and out of direct patient care in hospital or community settings and into a day-long professional regional or state event. These activities included a state nurses' association convention, Sigma Theta Tau local chapter Research Day, and a legislative/political nursing conference.

In all these experiences, a puzzling personal reflection surfaced. I dearly wanted the nursing profession to be "displayed" in all its goodness, energy, and power. Furthermore, I think I wanted the students to see this and only this display. It was almost as if I sought to "show off" nursing.

In reality, however, students' perception of these activities was mixed. After attendance at a recent conference, one student exclaimed, "It was so amazing to see how excited and motivated everyone was about their beloved profession. I know I'm joining a great profession!" Yet, after the same experience, another student bemoaned, "I felt a little shocked that only about 200–300 nurses were present. I would have loved to see more nurses represented. I felt there was a generation gap; very seasoned nurses and very fresh nurses or nursing students. It would have been nice to see younger/newer nurses."

Initially, these lights and shadows of professional nursing troubled me. But then I stepped back to rethink. In truth, if I view these professional socialization experiences the way I view clinical experiences, I should expect the strengths and limitations in them. After all, I readily see both the distinction as well as the blemishes in any other clinical experience. The challenge for me, then, is to help students learn to be leaders within a bumpy, less-than-perfect profession.

Teaching and learning about leadership and professionalism and influencing change in this way remind me of Allen and Allen's premise in *Escaping the Endless Adolescence* (2009). They caution that keeping teens in a bubble with helicopter, overnurturing parenting results in young adults incapable of taking risks, finding meaning, and serving others. Hence, the adolescence is endless, with age 25 being the new age 15.

Similarly, we must avoid presenting only an idealized view of the profession to the students. As we design clinical experiences to help students learn various professional roles, including nursing leadership, we must create candid and above-board scaffolds. The assistance itself, the scaffold that we provide, demands thoughtfulness as it also becomes part of the learning and the discovery. That is, it is not only what happens as a result of the scaffold—it is the scaffold in its own right that fosters learning.

We must be honest in who we are as a profession; only then will students understand challenges more completely and design their own strategies more effectively. As one insightful student noted, "As seasoned nurses leave the workforce the younger nurses must be able to step up and assume leadership of the profession."

Cheryl's Story: The Good, the Bad, and the Ugly

One of the joys of coordinating an ABSN program is the opportunity to work closely with the students across the entire curriculum. I am privileged to have a part in everything from planning the students' pre-program orientation to filing their final course grade so that they can graduate. I also teach courses in three of the program's four terms. This long view offers a perspective from which to see the gratifying successes as well as the dismaying failures we have had in the program.

One of our successes has been the incorporation of technology, such as high-fidelity human patient simulators, into several courses in the program. I like saying that we have created a "simulation-rich" program. From the first term to the last we use simulated patient care experiences for learning physical assessment, clinical reasoning, patient teaching, and care management using unfolding scenarios. This makes me proud of our motivated faculty and our supportive Skills Lab team. Benner, Sutphen, Leonard, and Day (2010), while acknowledging that more research is needed on the benefits and limitations of simulation, noted that pedagogies that engage students "offer a means to integrate the kind of learning that today's nurses need for practice" (p. 162).

For me, one of the most disappointing failures to date stemmed from an attempt to equip the students with the latest web-based learning tools. I had the best of intentions. Knowing that they would be pressured for time I calculated that electronic and web-based learning resources would give students access whenever and wherever they were connected to the Internet. No longer would they need to carry heavy textbooks and spend extra time on campus viewing assigned media.

Part of my brilliant plan was to pilot the use of electronic textbooks and access to online streaming videos demonstrating physical assessment techniques. Imagine my disappointment when students reported problems with both products. The electronic textbooks were not user-friendly; they took a long time to search, much longer than it took to flip the pages of a textbook. Additionally, the videos took forever to load and even longer to view given the frequent hiccups in the video stream. The students were dissatisfied with both products.

We contacted the sales and technical support staff of the company from whom we had purchased the online video product, ultimately learning that the company had contracted out maintenance of its server to a firm located in the Netherlands. It turned out that the subcontracting firm had been having some trouble with their server! The tools intended to equip the students for maximum mobility in their learning ended up slowing them down. Purchase of that online video series has not been required since.

Finally, we have had one "failure" that became an opportunity for a student to demonstrate success. The failure was in our development of learning assignments. Faculty tried to make every learning assignment meet a clearly identified learning goal. We wanted enough assignments to enable students to demonstrate learning but not so many that they were unnecessarily duplicative and "busy work" (Cangelosi, 2007b; Hamner & Bentley, 2007).

We realized that there was not yet a lean and meaningful core of learning assignments when Sarah presented us with a two-page list of each assignment in every course in the program, gleaned from course syllabi and organized by assignment type. For example, "Sarah's List" showed us we were assigning more care plans than most students needed to demonstrate understanding of the clinical decision-making process. In addition, there were several assignments that involved interviewing friends and/or family members. Students' ability to complete those assignments was contingent on being able to arrange interviews around their rigid class and clinical schedules. Lastly, assignments did not build well on each other. For example, students were assigned to read a research article and write a basic annotated bibliography two terms after they demonstrated the ability to read and carefully critique research.

Teacher failure thus opened the door for student success; Sarah became an agent of change. Practicing some of what she had learned, she carefully collected data and submitted them with a respectful request to evaluate the need for each assignment. Ultimately, our failure coupled with Sarah's response is an example of the engagement, dialog, and exchange called for in Kleiman's Humanistic Teaching Model (2007). The "ah-ha" for me: even a failure can be a success when it becomes an opportunity for students to shine.

Our Final Story: Surviving, Sustaining, and Succeeding

Our final story shifts from an "ah-ha" moment to an "ahhh" experience. It is here that we can rest, assured by each others' support and sustained by each others' glow.

This "ahhh" experience is about us, perhaps more intimately than our earlier stories. We remember Parker Palmer's approach to learning "on the slant" (2004, p. 92). He described the process of exploring "soul truth" indirectly because it is so powerful. Palmer maintained that "we must invite, not command, the soul to speak" (p. 92). For us, our support of each other is soul truth and we have only begun to honor the invitation. This is our final story, "on the slant."

Our faculty experience emerges from intensity and letting go. Just as the demands of the program mean intensity for the students, they also mean intensity for us. Haughtiness notwithstanding, it may be impossible to grasp the program's stress until you have lived in the thick of it.

In this intensity, we let some things go. To be precise, we have sacrificed some aspects of family and other personal life. And, to be honest, this sacrifice sometimes has broken hearts and anguished spirits.

In this intensity, time splits seconds. As we check off one task on our to-do list, there are 15 more clamoring to take its place—pleading for instant completion. When issues arise, there is little room to breathe and little time to consult with colleagues, as they must be addressed within the moment. Students need an answer on the spot; as adult learners, they learn from an urgency perspective—they are already moving on to the next problem, working toward the next goal. Our response determines where they go and what they do in the next 24 hours. We cannot say, "I'll talk with the other course faculty to see how we might handle this," because that might not be for several days or a week. And between now and then, there will be three eight-hour class days and two eight-hour clinical days, two papers due, and an exam to take online. Yikes .... we could never wait that long! As Melissa concluded, "I just dealt with it." And, of course, Melissa knew that we would support her.

In this intensity, there is a need for brevity. We cannot spend hours describing the issue or writing pages about options and "best choice." We have created a culture where a few words suffice. For example, as a faculty team, we all know that Shannon will be challenged in the hospital, as she prefers community nursing care and will likely excel there as an RN. So, in our discussion about Shannon's success in the next hospital clinical rotation, CeCelia instantly offers scaffolding strategies to help her succeed, such as priority lists, clinical contracts, and scheduled meeting times through the shift. We know the students and we know each other. Most of the time, we just know.

In this intensity, we survive because we also know that others "have our back" because they too are equally committed to this endeavor. Yet, this is not merely about someone "taking a bullet for me; it is about someone picking me up when I stumble and hearing me blow off steam when I must." It is Melissa's continual thinking ahead; she has "saved my butt more times than I'll ever know because she is such a plan-full person." It is also Cheryl "fielding my calls, day or night" to make certain that I am not repeating content, but also ensuring that I am not omitting something essential.

Still, living with this intensity is more than survival; we live with this intensity in success. Our success grows from a detailed and rich relationship with each other that forms from teaching in the trenches together, closely, month after month. Admittedly, we have all been in other courses where palpable power struggles shriveled course development and, thus, diminished student learning. But our relationship in the ABSN program builds on alliance. Also, it is more than just a statement of courtesy—a "how are you?" in the school corridor—it is "CeCelia's genuine concern for me as a person." Our relationships are carried by compassion and held in trust over time. Just as the students bond with one another, this program also brings us together in profound ways. Humanism, then, is also a commitment by teacher to teacher, and not merely a commitment by teacher to student.

In this business, it is perhaps because we all see ourselves as learners with the students that we have created an open circle of discovery. CeCelia's gentle "on the other hand" reminds us of the complexity of issues and calls us to engage in respectful discourse. In her mirthful, sober Cheryl-ese, she "holds our feet to the fire" in the decisions we make and the reasons as to why we make them. As constructivists, therefore, our relationships scaffold our learning; they help us notice in new ways and connect ideas in fresh patterns.

Our success also grows from learning with the students over most of the 12-month program. In the traditional program, teaching assignments often push and pull us in and out of semesters over a three-year professional program, and we may only see students in one slice of their baccalaureate experience. For instance, we may see students as first semester juniors and then never see what they have learned by program's end. In this traditional program model, we spend endless energy learning about students as students learn about nursing and learn about us. The next semester, we all begin anew.

However, in the ABSN program we teach and learn with students across their academic career as they develop into professional nurses. As a result, we reap the benefits of our investment.

Finally, our success grows because we live on the edge of our comfort, on the margin of our tribe (in this situation, "tribe" refers to teaching philosophy, educator techniques, communication style, etc.). In living on the edge, not only have we grown in self-knowledge but we have also grown in knowledge of each other. In their qualitative study over several years, with over 100 individuals who had sustained commitments to work on behalf of the common good (Parks Daloz, Keen, Keen, & Daloz Parks, 1996), researchers discovered a "constructive, enlarging engagement with the other" (p. 63). This engagement involved seeing both resemblance and difference. The researchers contended that, "seeing resemblance in difference does not mean blurring the distinctions that constitute the integrity of the particular, nor denying differences that are experienced as difficult or repugnant. It means that one has recognized a shared resonance of spirit in our common life …" (p. 77).

Through our stories we have attempted to put "flesh on the bones" of adult theory, constructivism, and humanism. In addition, we have used the literature and educational theories to illuminate our experiences. It is this praxis where theory and literature meet the teacher, which sustains teaching excellence and enhances student learning.

CHALLENGES, STRATEGIES, RECOMMENDATIONS: PARTING WORDS

In this praxis, too, the teacher confronts challenges, explores strategies, and selects from an array of recommendations. The primary challenges emerge from the fast pace of the curriculum resulting in a compressed time for teaching and an intense time for learning.

Not only do we face these challenges on a "big picture" program planning and curricular design level, but we also meet them on a daily, moment-to-moment level. For example, we create alternatives when a professor unexpectedly needs a medical leave of absence during a time when she was expected to teach 30 hours of specialized class content over the next three weeks. Or, a clinical agency forbids students from documenting during a three-week clinical experience because of its transition to an electronic medical record system. Yet, this clinical experience comprises a significant number of clinical hours in the first month of a term. As there is so little cushion in the accelerated program—limited staffing buffers and razor-thin class or clinical alternatives—the challenges escalate.

For us, meeting these challenges requires strategies deeply rooted in our values and beliefs. First, we value each other's strengths and lean on them heavily. Second, we believe that a team is stronger and more effective than what we could do individually. This team is committed to students' learning and augmenting each other's talents.

We offer our recommendations, not as a "to-do" list, but only from a place of learning, self-reflection, and near-misses. Day after day, we remind ourselves and each other that the students are adult learners. Further, we view ourselves as learners too, adopting an attitude of humble curiosity as we revise assignments, evaluation methods, course organization, and the curricular program. In this collaborative venture, the students are our finest teachers.

Several other recommendations have upheld our teaching and learning. Acknowledging the change in identity that second-degree students experience as they become novices again is critical. We deliberately emphasize reflection and professional formation in this transition. In truth, because we concede the lights and shadows of the nursing profession, we join students in their reflection, their formation, and their quest to make it better. Once again, the students are our finest teachers.

In telling our stories, then, we are learning the value of truthful and courageous self-reflection. Sometimes we listen ardently to student voices. Sometimes students need to listen to us. And sometimes, despite the strength of students' resolve and the worthy meaning of their message, we do not hear them. Yet, in the midst of this intensity, we are beginning to discover the essence of faculty excellence.

REFERENCES

Allen, J., & Allen, C. W. (2009). *Escaping the endless adolescence: How we can help our teenagers grow up before they grow old.* New York: Ballantine.

Benner, P., Sutphen, M., Leonard, V., & Day, L. (2010). *Educating nurses, a call for radical transformation.* San Francisco: Jossey-Bass.

Cangelosi, P. R. (2007a). Accelerated second-degree baccalaureate nursing programs: What is the significance of clinical instructors? *Journal of Nursing Education, 46*(9), 400–405.

Cangelosi, P. R. (2007b). Voices of graduates from second-degree baccalaureate nursing programs. *Journal of Professional Nursing, 23*(2), 91–97.

Cangelosi, P. R., & Moss, M. M. (2010). Voices of faculty of second-degree baccalaureate nursing students. *Journal of Nursing Education, 49*(3), 137–142.

Clark, C. S. (2005). Transforming nursing education: A partnership social system for alignment with philosophies of care. *International Journal of Nursing Education Scholarship, 2*(1), 1–17.

DeSimone, B. B. (2006). Curriculum design to promote the critical thinking of accelerated bachelor's degree nursing students. *Nurse Educator, 31*(5), 213–217.

Ediger, M. (2006). Present day philosophies of education. *Journal of Instructional Psychology, 33*(3), 179–182.

Hamner, J. B., & Bentley, R. (2007). Lessons learned from 12 years of teaching second-degree BSN students. *Nurse Educator, 32*(3), 126–129.

Hydo, S. K., Marcyjanik, D. L., Zorn, C. R., & Hooper, N. M. (2007). Art as a scaffolding teaching strategy in baccalaureate nursing education. *International Journal of Nursing Education Scholarship, 4*(1), 1–13.

Kleiman, S. (2007). Revitalizing the humanistic imperative in nursing education. *Nursing Education Perspectives, 28*(4), 209–213.

Knowles, M. S., Holton, E. F., III, & Swanson, R. A. (2005). *The adult learner: The definitive classic in adult education and human resource development* (6th ed.). New York: Elsevier.

Lindsey, P. (2009). Starting an accelerated baccalaureate nursing program: Challenges and opportunities for creative education innovations. *Journal of Nursing Education, 48*(5), 279–281.

Lockwood, S., Walker, C. A., & Tilley, D. S. (2009). Faculty perceptions of an accelerated baccalaureate nursing program. *Journal of Nursing Education, 48*(7), 406–410.

Miklancie, M., & Davis, T. (2005). The second-degree accelerated program as an innovative education strategy: New century, new chapter, new challenge. *Nursing Education Perspectives, 26*(5), 291–293.

Murray, T. A. (2007). Expanding educational capacity through an innovative practice-education partnership. *Journal of Nursing Education, 46*(7), 330–333.

Palmer, P. J. (2004). *A hidden wholeness: The journey toward an undivided life.* San Francisco, CA: Jossey-Bass.

Parks Daloz, L. A., Keen, C. H., Keen, J. P., & Daloz Parks, S. (1996). *Common fire: Leading lives of commitment in a complex world.* Boston: Beacon Press.

Raines, D. A. (2006). CAN-Care: An innovative model of practice-based learning. *International Journal of Nursing Education Scholarship, 3*(1), 1–17.

Rodgers, M., Burson, J., & Kirschling, J. (2004). Developing an accelerated BSN program: One college's experience. *Nursing Leadership Forum, 9*(1), 18–22.

Safstrom, C. A. (2003). Teaching otherwise. *Studies in Philosophy and Education, 22,* 19–29.

Schreier, A. M., Peery, A. I., & McLean, C. B. (2009). An integrative curriculum for accelerated nursing education programs. *Journal of Nursing Education, 48*(5), 282–285.

Suliman, W. A. (2006). Critical thinking and learning styles of students in conventional and accelerated programmes. *International Nursing Review, 53,* 73–79.

Suplee, P. D., & Glasgow, M. E. (2008). Curriculum innovation in an accelerated BSN program: The ACE model. *International Journal of Nursing Education Scholarship, 5*(1), 1–13.

Utley-Smith, Q., Phillips, B., & Turner, K. (2007). Avoiding socialization pitfalls in accelerated second-degree nursing education: The returning-to-school syndrome model. *Journal of Nursing Education, 46*(9), 423–426.

Vandeveer, M. (2009). From teaching to learning, theoretical foundations. In D. M. Billings & J. A. Halstead (Eds.), *Teaching in nursing. A guide for faculty* (pp. 189–226). St. Louis, MO: Saunders Elsevier.

Vinal, D. F., & Whitman, N. (1994). The second time around: Nursing as a second degree. *Journal of Nursing Education, 33*(1), 37–39.

Vygotsky, L. S. (1962). In E. Hanfmann & G. Vakar (Eds. & Transl.), *Thought and language*. Cambridge: Massachusetts Institute of Technology Press.

Vygotsky, L. S. (1978). In M. Cole (Ed.), *Mind in society: The development of higher psychological processes*. Cambridge, MA: Harvard University Press.

Walker, C., Tilley, D. S., Lockwood, S., & Walker, M. B. (2008). An innovative approach to accelerated baccalaureate education. *Nursing Education Perspectives, 29*(6), 347–352.

Walker, J. T., Martin, T. M., Haynie, L., Norwood, A., White, J., & Grant, L. (2007). Preferences for teaching methods in a baccalaureate nursing program: How second-degree and traditional students differ. *Nursing Education Perspectives, 28*(5), 246–250.

Watson, J. (2000). A new paradigm of curriculum development. In E. O. Bevis & J. Watson (Eds.), *Toward a caring curriculum: A new pedagogy for nursing* (pp. 37–49). Sudbury, MA: Jones and Bartlett.

Weitzel, M. L., & McCahon, C. P. (2008). Stressors and supports for baccalaureate nursing students completing an accelerated program. *Journal of Professional Nursing, 24*(2), 85–89.

Leadership in Accelerated Nursing Education

Chapter

7

Leading and Inspiring a Shared Vision

Lin Zhan, Linda P. Finch, Shirleatha Lee, and Jill Dapremont

*A*ccelerated nursing education is an innovative approach to address the needs of preparing professional nursing workforce. Academic leaders in nursing are called not only to design, implement, and evaluate accelerated programs but also to lead and inspire a shared vision. Good leaders possess qualities and characteristics necessary to make things happen. It is essential for academic leaders to be visionary and have the ability to motivate and inspire others toward a desired goal (Clark, 2004; Fowler, 2011). The ability to lead requires providing a clear vision and a clear understanding of the direction of the organization and its ultimate goals. A clear vision grants a sense of what the organization "hopes to become" or "aspires to be." The vision also enhances organizational successes by inspiring and unifying individuals in their efforts (Quigley, 1994; Slack, Orife, & Anderson, 2010).

A vision is the foundation for trust and commitment in the organization, and a shared vision as shared pictures of the future fosters genuine commitment and enrollment by all involved (Senge, 2006). While much research examines how leaders effectively inspire a unified vision that provides direction to followers, the ability to share vision is complex and challenging. This chapter thus examines the key elements of inspired leadership, development of a shared vision and articulation in an accelerated nursing program, and challenges in leading and inspiring a shared vision.

KEY ELEMENTS OF INSPIRED LEADERSHIP

Effective and inspired leadership is complex and comprises multiple components. With challenging and changing health environments, including academic settings, those in leadership positions realize that being successful requires a leader to commit to a shared vision. Leaders envision exciting possibilities and enlist others in a shared view of the future, which is the attribute that most distinguishes leaders from nonleaders. Research by Kouzes and Posner (2008) revealed that leaders most often struggle with communicating an image of the future, a vision that draws others in and resonates with what others see and feel. Thus, the only visions that take hold are shared visions that evolve when leaders listen closely to others, appreciate their hopes, and attend to their needs (Kouzes and Posner, 2008). A shared vision requires team effort, fosters mutual trust and respect, motivates and inspires, creates a collaborative culture, develops common threads, promotes faculty participation, and brings problem-resolves.

Mutual Trust and Respect

An effective leader is admired and respected. The leader creates an environment that nurtures a sense of trust and respect between and among followers. Trust is built when the leaders clearly communicate what they stand for, what they value, what they want, what they hope for, and what they are willing to do or not to do (Kouzes and Posner, 2008). This approach can be risky, as it may disclose leaders' vulnerability; yet, leaders' willingness to take risks allows others to reciprocate. Building trust requires efforts made by leaders to listen to and be sensitive to people's needs and interests. Trust in an academic setting is about reliability, focus, and constancy. Reliability is dependability as defined by focus and constancy (Tecker, Frankel, & Meyer, 2002). To earn respect from followers, leaders must be willing to be respectful of others, which may not be based solely on what one says but more on what one does. Followers carefully observe their leader for display of the ethical principles and values to which they ascribe. The most respected leaders not only talk about their ethical values and principles but also reflect these in their daily practice. Integrity is an internally consistent framework of ethical values and principles. Leaders with integrity show honesty, truthfulness, ethical consciousness, fairness, and justice. By "walking the talk," leaders are more likely to create a culture of mutual trust and respect that strengthens his/her ability to motivate and inspire a shared vision.

Motivates and Inspires

Leaders inspire a vision and motivate others to follow it. What leadership is needed to effectively motivate and inspire others? Transformational leadership, originally introduced by Burns (1978) and later elaborated by Bass (1985), described transformational leaders as flexible and adaptable to change in challenging environments. The transformational leadership theory suggests that enhanced motivation and empowerment of followers be essential to achieve success (Avolio, Zhu, Koh, & Bahtia, 2004). A transformational leader envisions the future and inspires others to commit to achieving the vision through positive motivation, enthusiasm, and integrity (Avolio et al., 2004). In practice, a transformation leader is open to new ideas; inquires about thoughts, beliefs, and feelings; encourages synergy; and fosters a shared vision.

While transformational leadership supports motivating and inspiring followers, it is important to understand that different situations may require different approaches of leadership. For example, novice faculty, new to teaching or to an academic setting, may require more oversight, mentoring, and direction than seasoned faculty. Additionally, some faculty may require more motivation than others. Therefore, it is important for leaders to be familiar with the faculty and have a good understanding of their needs and their own visions (Clark, 2004). While each individual is different, leaders should acknowledge individual differences yet utilize the appropriate transformational leadership to motivate and inspire faculty for a shared vision.

Collaborative Culture

In an academic setting, collaboration is necessary, as no single person can fulfill the mission of the institution. Collaborations such as purposefully built relationships are necessary to achieve shared outcomes. In daily practice, effective collaboration or teamwork results in high performance and improved efficiency as evidenced by people who share information, listen to each other's ideas, exchange resources, respond to each other's request through positive interdependence, and provide support to resolve problems. Collaborative leadership is needed to foster a culture of collaboration. To create a collaborative culture, leaders should possess critical skills and capability to: (a) assess the context or environment for collaboration, (b) lead peer problem-solving, to build broad-based involvement, (c) create clarity by defining shared values and aspirations, (d) share power and influence by developing synergy of people to accomplish goals, and (e) develop people by mentoring and coaching. Collaboration involves people working together even with different skill sets and backgrounds. Therefore, it is important for academic leaders to give time to members so that they become acquainted, are able to discuss collaborative goals, and have time to work together. Supporting teamwork promotes a sense of unity and prevents member isolation. In building and working in a collaborative culture, leaders and members openly discuss values, beliefs, and commitments that all lead to shared vision (Leithwood & Poplin, 1992).

Collaborative leadership represents a paradigm shift in which people work together to lead an organization forward (Rickard and Harding, 2000). In academic settings, collaborative leadership helps create an environment of shared governance and enables faculty to be a part of vision development. Communicating thoughts and ideas connects and motivates individuals and increases commitment (Kolzow, 1999). The process of shared vision development helps produce positive outcomes in the work environment (Schultz, 2011), including feeling a sense of ownership that transitions people from accepting the organization as "theirs" owned by others, to "ours"—owned by all involved (Senge, 2006). Collaborative leadership encourages people to be an intricate part of moving forward to achieve the established goals.

Common Threads

To inspire a shared vision, individuals' dreams, aspirations, or personal visions need to be identified. In the process of imaging the ideal and intuiting the future, common threads can be found and built as the foundation for a shared vision. For example, member of faculty may share a vision for students' success. It is not unusual for nurse educators to personally envision students successfully completing the nursing program, passing the licensure exam, and entering the nursing profession. From the moment students take their course, faculty strive to provide them with opportunities to acquire the knowledge and skills necessary to assume the role of a professional nurse. When graduates achieve high NCLEX-RN pass rates, faculty often share the excitement of this achievement. Thus, working to attain high NCLEX-RN pass rates is a common thread among nursing faculty. In schools of nursing, common threads, such as student retention and graduation, establish connections among faculty and leaders and become both personal and organizational visions. Often, the school of nursing envisions creating a center of excellence in teaching, research, and service/practice. These three broad areas serve as a framework for faculty tenure and promotion criteria, and thus, become a common thread of excellence that individual faculty and the organization strive toward attaining. So again, a key element in sharing a vision is to define outcomes important to all organizational members who collectively work toward accomplishing the defined outcomes. In this process of working toward a shared vision, both leaders and faculty have a personal connection with the organization vision that, not only increases the likelihood of successful organizational outcomes but also heightens the individual investment and development in an organization (Quigley, 1994).

Faculty Participation

A shared vision involves a broad-based participation. In the school of nursing, it is imperative for faculty, students, and staff participation in developing the vision, deciding core values, and formulating strategic goals. The role of the leaders is to clearly articulate organizational goals and objectives. When people are aware of the expectations, they can make a plan and move toward their personal and professional goals. Leaders' expectations should be ambitious but reasonable, allowing faculty feedback and involvement in problem solving, helps develop further commitment to vision, and inspires them to strive for excellence in purpose (Leithwood & Poplin, 1992). Shared governance is an approach that supports faculty participation. Forms of the shared governance may involve faculty-led committees, faculty organizations, faculty-led task forces or ad hoc committees, and organizational bylaws. Participatory leadership is needed to encourage faculty participation since it allows power sharing and empowers faculty to participate in decision-making related to quality education.

Improved Problem-Solving

Within an environment of mutual trust and respect, which motivates and inspires, promotes a collaborative culture, identifies common threads, and promotes broad-based participation, problems are solved in a more efficient way. In an inspiring environment, members of faculty are allowed opportunities to freely discuss problems and determine ways to solve problems. Faculty members focus on finding options, solutions, tactics, and/or strategies to solve problems rather than complaining about the problems. Open collaboration allows for seeking alternative perspectives and generates optional ways for handing problems within the broad organizational framework (Leithwood & Poplin, 1992). Leaders promote these open discussions, minimize preconceived solutions, and are obliged to new strategies and approaches. Data are collected that aid in problem analyses. Transformational leaders realize that grass-root-driven decision-making is a more positive approach to resolve problems than a top-down approach.

VISION DEVELOPMENT AND ARTICULATION WITHIN AN ACCELERATED NURSING PROGRAM

Developing and articulating a shared vision often begins with the strategic planning processes. Strategic planning is a formal and critical analysis of the past and future and can be utilized to develop both short- and long-term goals (Lozier & Chittipeddi, 1986). To be effective, strategic planning should be knowledge based, inclusive, and future oriented. Involvement of all levels of employees in the strategic planning process supports the foundation of a shared vision.

The process of developing a vision reflective of accelerated nursing educational programming should include five characteristics: (1) who you are, (2) what you do, (3) where you are going, (4) how you will know when you get there, and (5) what are people saying about your organization (Yokl, 2011, p. 52). When describing "who you are" (p. 52), think of what your organization represents. Asking simple questions about the school of nursing and its goals while seeking faculty input can be beneficial (Cheneski, 2011). Does an accelerated program have a special niche or configuration that makes it different from others, such as offering a solely online program or weekend classes? Open dialog about where the school of nursing currently and, in particular, an accelerated nursing program is and where it would like to be in the future is essential. When this process is started, all members of the organization should be invited to participate so that they feel included and their voices are heard, and the process is necessary to ensure "buy in" of a new accelerated program in nursing. While multiple meetings are never easy, they may be necessary during the process of establishing common themes and goals when considering and planning for accelerated nursing education programming.

Next, examine, "what you do" (p. 52). Think about the overall purpose of one's organization. Is an accelerated nursing program focused on producing nursing leaders, preparing nurses to enter graduate school, or meeting the health care needs of the community? The foundation of "what you do" should be aligned with the mission of an overall institution and program. Therefore, it is important to have a clear understanding of what differentiates a mission from a vision. The mission describes the overall purpose of an organization, while the vision describes the future of the organization. Most universities have many departments and each department has to define its specific purpose within the university. Therefore, when developing the vision of the accelerated nursing program, one should ensure that it is aligned with the mission and vision of the department and the institution.

In describing "where you are going" (p. 52), the first recognition is to focus on the goal, the future, what is to be accomplished, and the aspiration for tomorrow. There is no expectation that is too big or too small. Personal visions of individual faculty can emerge as centralized themes that are priority ranked as low, moderate, or high (Kolzow, 1999). This process of developing a vision statement helps to facilitate that all voices are heard and allows everyone to listen, discuss, and agree on common threads in support of the values of each individual as well as the value of the institution. Once a tentative vision statement is developed, the draft should be presented to the organization for more discussion and revision, if necessary. This type of communication process promotes exchange of ideas and energizes the organization (Grohar-Murray & Langan, 2011). The information collected assists in the development of the final shared vision statement which should be brief, positive, easy to understand, and achievable (Cheneski, 2011).

Following the development of the vision statement, one question to be answered is "How you will know when you get there" (p. 52). Vision is an *ideal* and purposefully creates a gap to inspire and motivate people to work collectively and individually toward that ideal (Kouzes and Posner, 2009). In the process, an organization develops a mission statement and a strategic plan with a defined timeframe. Methods of measurement are used to determine if the mission and strategies are met. In a nursing program, some measurements occur via student evaluations, alumni surveys, and/or the assessment by community leaders. Critical for evaluation are the necessary educational resources (human, fiscal, and physical) that enable an organization to reach its strategic goals. Each organization should select the method(s) that best gauges its success and assists in staying on task to fulfill its mission. Established benchmarks and measurements allow for corrective actions or reevaluation of the mission as necessary. When a shared vision is crafted, any gap needs analysis, which provides information used to design, implement, and evaluate needed faculty development, educational recourses, academic policies and procedures, and service to interests of the community. Motivating faculty through training, continued education, and/or counseling, along with providing faculty with the necessary resources, are essential elements in fulfilling the mission and sustain a shared vision.

Lastly, examining "what are people saying about your organization" (p. 52) helps to determine if the vision is embraced. Are faculty, staff, and students excited about their accomplishments? The organization's members should listen to what people say about the organization, including people inside and outside the organization within the community. This communication is essential because it supports inclusion and helps the vision continue to inspire people (Kolzow, 1999). Determining whether the feedback is positive or negative and if there are any consistent themes helps assist in sustaining a shared vision.

Formulating ideas and writing a shared vision statement is multifaceted. Deciding when to formulate the vision (i.e., strategic planning), obtaining past and present knowledge about the organization, and determining how to best organize faculty to ensure an inclusive process are all important elements. Methods to achieve these tasks may vary across institutions. However, the foundation of a shared vision remains the same; it is the combination of many personal visions. The end result is a vision statement that is clear, concise, coherent, achievable, and accepted by all. The shared vision is a source of motivation and inspiration for both leaders and followers to achieve organizational goals.

CHALLENGES IN VISION DEVELOPMENT AND FULFILLMENT

The nursing profession has a rich and deep past. Many faculties have become accustomed to educating students in a traditional manner and are indoctrinated and support traditional programs. Therefore, developing a shared vision that embraces an innovative approach to teaching in an accelerated program can spark uneasiness and debate. Innovation requires use of outsight and insight, inseparable concepts if the leaders challenge the status quo and make necessary changes. Outsight means to stay in touch with a world of trends, issues, treats, and possibilities. For example, outsight followed by open dialog provides discussion opportunities between leaders and faculty, with analysis of differences in educating nursing students in an accelerated program in comparison with the traditional model. In addition, core values and common goals in nursing education are identified and supported by the faculty, as these values and goals can be integrated in the accelerated nursing program.

Although the leader may have a clear vision and is supported by many of the faculty, all faculty may not be in agreement. Again, many likely have past experiences where organizational changes were mandated from leadership without input or buy in from those obligated to implement the changes. As a result, faculty and staff may half-heartedly execute the necessary changes. They may also speak negatively about the process, hindering the success of the new method and leading to the gradual return of the status quo. It is not surprising that some faculty may oppose the progression to an accelerated program despite continued efforts to inspire them in that direction. Therefore, it is important for leaders to prepare for implementing major changes, including new type of programming such as an accelerated option so that these negative reactions and resistance may be minimized. There are several mechanisms by which the leader can manage faculty resistance.

First, the leader should ensure that faculty and staff are aware of the plan to implement the accelerated nursing program in the initial stages. Unexpected changes can be shocking and may receive resistance. Willingness to share ideas, plans, benefits, and possible challenges for the implementation of the accelerated program gives faculty a chance to explore decision-making possibilities and contribute to the decision-making process. When communicating a plan for new programming, relevant data are needed, such as needs assessment of the market, critical resources, and profession. As faculties contribute to the processes they become a part of program development and are less likely to resist change.

Secondly, identifying how day-to-day decisions within the organization contribute to the vision. This level of communication helps individual faculty to understand each part of the plan and how each piece works together to obtain the ultimate goal. Having this level of understanding allows individuals to identify the importance of their contribution to the goal. For example, if a committee is formed to hire new faculty and these faculty may instruct within the accelerated nursing program, make this connection. Let the faculty that serve on the committee know the importance and value of their service commitment and how they are an intricate part of achieving the ultimate goal. This will help faculty have a better understanding of their role in developing the accelerated nursing program. It will also help them to identify the importance of their roles. Next, faculty should be given the opportunity to receive additional education and training so that they can participate in the implementation of the accelerated nursing program. This empowers individuals to perform to the greatest extent of their potential. It can also decrease resistance, because members of faculty are informed, engaged, and capable to deal with newness if applicable for teaching in the accelerated program.

Open and constant communication among leaders and faculty is essential when implementing an accelerated nursing program. A shared vision for an accelerated nursing program will excite and motivate faculty whose ideas and concerns are valued and respected. Leaders listen thoughtfully and provide careful consideration to faculty concerns that provide motivation to achieve the organizational goals. Much of communication is nonverbal and how one communicates with faculty and staff can build or impair relationships (Clark, 2004). So, if leaders do not communicate with and listen to faculty in the program development stages, a key element may be missed. It is difficult to convey a vision and implement change when faculty are not aware of the vision or any upcoming changes. Therefore, the vision is less likely to be fulfilled.

To enhance support of the shared vision, it is important that timelines are effectively communicated to reduce unexpected surprises. If there is an anticipated date the accelerated program will be initiated, the timeline should be shared with the faculty well in advance. This will allow the faculty time to prepare for the upcoming change and reduce resistance to the implementation of the new program.

Lastly, sometimes followers are reluctant to change because they sense that things are fine as they are. Therefore, leaders should generate a sense of importance that should be identified in the initial planning stages. Several examples may include a change in the student population that the community serves, a decline in students enrolled in the traditional nursing program, or possibly the accelerated nursing program will be the first or only program in the region. Thus, the articulated vision must be supported by evidence of need. The leader should describe how the organization could grow and build as a result of the implementation of the accelerated nursing program (Grohar-Murray & Langan, 2011). A sense of importance should describe why it is urgent and necessary to achieve this goal. The leader should not only detail the benefits of developing an accelerated nursing program, but also the drawbacks of not doing so.

It can also be a challenge for the leader if the faculty gets off track in the development of the accelerated program. The leader must be aware that this can occur, especially if new issues or problems arise that derails focus from the vision. The leader must be prepared to take corrective action and get individuals back on target to reach organizational goals (King, 2011). Therefore, it is important that the leader stays on target, as well. If someone or a group of individuals lose focus on the vision, the leader guides them back in the right direction using effective communication and meaningful insight (King, 2011), stressing the importance of each individual, and providing necessary education or training as needed (Grohar-Murray & Langan, 2011).

A vision to implement the accelerated nursing program into the organizational curriculum requires the leader to anticipate challenges. It is important to develop a shared vision that is reflective of the personal and philosophical beliefs of faculty. However, it is helpful to understand that 100% buy-in is sought but not guaranteed. Therefore, it is leaders that make faculty being aware of the plan early, identify day-to-day contributions to the long-term goal, communicate effectively, generate a sense of importance, stay on target, and anticipate faculty resistance as a possible challenge to vision fulfillment.

SUMMARY

Visions are about future possibilities. Visions articulate standards of excellence. A shared vision engages, empowers, and enables all involved to face challenges, strive for a higher level of excellence, and collaborate to accomplish shared goals. Effective leadership is called to inspire, motivate, and support faculty, staff, and students in an ever-changing educational and healthcare environment. Personal characteristics, beliefs, values, and ethics of individuals are all attributes that make each leader unique (Clark, 2004). However, it is important that leaders examine their leadership style to ensure that it is accepting of collaborative leadership and shared vision development. This encompasses being inclusive of all members of the organization in the development of the vision.

The accelerated nursing program is growing in response to the shortage of nursing workforce. To develop and sustain an accelerated program, academic leaders and faculty can benefit from developing a shared vision reflective of organizational goals, personal and philosophical beliefs of the faculty, and ideality for the pursuit of excellence. The shared vision inspires all toward involvement for the betterment of nursing education.

Change invites resistance. A moment of chaos, imbalance, and uncertainty becomes a primary resource of creativity. Therefore, it is essential that leaders keep positive attitudes throughout the process (Machiavelli, 2011), and prepare for challenges that may arise during or after the development of the vision. Maintaining an open line of communication is one of the most critical elements needed to stay on track and resolve challenges during this process. Further, faculty are supplied with the necessary resources and training to overcome any barriers in goal attainment.

The development of a shared vision to achieve more desirable outcomes has the ability to motivate and inspire followers to achieve organizational goals. It is the role of a leader to guide followers to develop and successfully fulfill the organization's shared vision. The organization's success is rooted in the vision that voices the future of the accelerated nursing program. Faculty, staff, and students can move the organization forward by embracing a vision that contributes to the successful obtainment of organizational goals. It can also attract highly qualified faculty, staff, and students that are motivated by the goals of the organization. There are many benefits to developing a shared vision for an accelerated nursing program, among which lies the ability to energize, motivate, and inspire successful outcomes.

REFERENCES

Avolio, B., Zhu, W., Koh, W., & Bahtia, P. (2004). Transformational leadership and organizational commitment: Mediating role of psychological empowerment and moderating role of structural distance. *Journal of Organizational Behavior, 25*(8), 951–968.

Bass, B. M. (1985). *Leadership and performance beyond expectations.* New York: Free Press.

Burns, J. M. (1978). *Leadership.* New York: Harper & Row.

Cheneski, W. (2011). Creating a meaningful vision statement. *Modern Machine Shop, 83*(11), 34.

Clark, D. R. (2004). *Concepts of leadership.* Retrieved June 12, 2011 from http://www.nwlink.com/~donclark/leader/leadcon.html

Fowler, J. (2011). Effective leadership. *Nursing Management United Kingdom, 17*(9), 38.

Grohar-Murray, M. E., & Langan, J. (2011). *Leadership and Management in Nursing* (4th ed.). New Jersey: Prentice-Hall.

King, M. (2011). Leadership: Give direction. Retrieved June 12, 2011 from http://learnthis.ca/2009/01/leadership-give-direction/

Kolzow, D. (1999). A perspective on strategic planning: What's your vision? *Economic Development Review, 16*(2), 5–9.

Kouzes, J. M., & Posner, B. Z. (2008). *The Leadership Challenge: How to Keep Getting Extraordinary Things Done in Organizations* (4th ed.). Jossey-Bass Publisher.

Kouzes, J. M., & Posner, B. Z. (2009). *To lead, create a shared vision.* Cambridge: Harvard Business Review Press.

Leithwood, K. A., & Poplin, M. S. (1992) The move toward transformational leadership. *Educational Leadership, 49*(5), 8.

Lozier, G., & Chittipeddi, K. (1986). Issues management in strategic planning. *Research in Higher Education, 24*(1), 3–14.

Machiavelli, N. (2011). *National defense university strategic leadership and vision making: Vision and management of change.* Retrieved June 10, 2011 from http://www.au.af.mil/au/awc/awcgate/ndu/strat-ldr-dm/pt4ch19.html

Quigley, J. (1994). Vision: How leaders develop it, share it, and sustain it. *Business Horizons, 37*(5), 37–41.

Rickard, C., & Harding, M. (2000). Strategic planning: A defined vision to facilitate institutional change. *College and University, 75*(3), 3–6.

Schultz, D. (2011). Sharing leadership. *Leadership Excellence, 28*(2), 16–17.

Senge, P. (2006). *The fifth discipline.* New York: Currency & Doubleday.

Slack, F., Orife, J., & Anderson, F. (2010). Effects of commitment to corporate vision on employee satisfaction with their organization: An empirical study in the United States. *International Journal of Management, 27*(3), 421–436.

Tecker, G. H., Frankel, J. S., & Meyer, P. D. (2002). *The will to govern well: Knowledge, trust, and nimbleness.* Washington, DC: American Society of Association Executives.

Yokl, R. (2011). Crafting a vision to optimize supply chain success. *Healthcare Purchasing News, 35*(2), 52.

Continuous Quality Improvement: Achieving Excellence

Lin Zhan

INTRODUCTION

A ccelerated education in nursing has grown rapidly to address the nursing shortage and to provide career opportunities in the midst of financial downturn in the United States. Most accelerated nursing programs are designed to meet the needs of individuals who hold a baccalaureate degree in a field other than nursing. These programs often require previously completed college general education courses combined with an additional 11 to 18 months of nursing courses. Some programs are targeted for those who want to pursue an advanced nursing degree in a shorter timeframe, such as fast-track master's degree programs. To date, according to the American Association of Colleges of Nursing (AACN, 2010), 43 states plus the District of Columbia and Guam offer accelerated nursing programs. In 2009, there were 230 accelerated baccalaureate programs and 65 accelerated master's programs available at nursing schools nationwide. In addition, 33 new accelerated baccalaureate and six accelerated master's programs are in the planning stages.

As accelerated programs are growing, a critical question is asked: how can nursing ensure the high quality of these accelerated programs? Nursing education is accountable and responsible to prepare undergraduates for entering the nursing profession competently and/or assuming the role of advanced practice and leadership in an ever-changing health care environment. Equally demanding is for higher education to meet or exceed learner and program outcomes, such as student retention, graduation, employment, and achievement. Accelerated nursing programs must move quickly and nimbly to deal with the challenges at hand, from insuring high educational quality amid growing student enrollments to a fast-paced curriculum and budgetary constraints placed on educational resources. A practice of continuous quality improvement (CQI) is therefore essential to facilitate changes and to improve outcomes of accelerated nursing programs on an ongoing basis.

CONTINUOUS QUALITY IMPROVEMENT: HISTORICAL PERSPECTIVES

The concept of continuous quality improvement (CQI) originated in 1949, when Japan requested help from Dr. W. Edwards Deming, an American quality improvement expert, to increase productivity and enhance the postwar quality of life for its people. This led to the widespread acceptance of Deming's philosophy (1986) of continuous improvement and his cycle for an improvement model: plan-do-study-act (Walton, 1988). Major principles in Deming's cycle include developing vision, mission, and values while listening to customers and employees. Only then should action be taken. Leaders must be champions for quality improvement and providers of resources necessary to remove obstacles for process improvement. Management and employees communicate with each other the rationales and merits of using CQI. Benchmarking is developed to show and measure actual progress in quality improvement.

Quality improvement also has a long history in service sectors. Notably, Florence Nightingale (Carroll, 1992) pioneered nursing and reformed hospitals using observations of statistics such as "*polar-area diagrams*" to compare mortality and morbidity causes in military and civilian circumstances. Her innovation led to dramatic changes in nursing's and hospital administration's focus on patient safety and quality. For their part, Ernest Amory Codman and Edward Martin used measurement of end results to standardize the practice of surgery in a hospital. When measuring the level of the physician–patient interaction, Avedis Donabedian identified three approaches to assessment: outcome of care, process of care, and structure (including the attributes of care providers, settings, and arrangements) (Donabedian, 1989; Ulrich, 1992).

During the 1970s, the oft-referenced search for "*quality*" in education was partly due to the increased consumerism of students and their critique of the educational "product" in higher education (Downey, 2000). Learner-centered education has since been advocated. Not only have leaders in higher education been challenged to analyze complex issues and justify decisions that affect academic programs, budgets, faculty, staff, and students, but educators have also transferred CQI principles into the classroom to improve teaching effectiveness. Furthermore, CQI as a management strategy has been used to aid in decision making. Terms associated with CQI in higher education include: committed leadership, adoption and communication of CQI, benchmarking, employee (student) empowerment, process improvement, and measurement. CQI coincides with the overall improvement of the educational process to accomplish set objectives (Steyn, 2000; Vora, 2002).

CONTINUOUS QUALITY IMPROVEMENT: DEFINED

Quality improvement is a system approach to reduce or eliminate waste, rework, and losses in the production process (Business Dictionary, 2011). It is a management philosophy. Underlying quality improvement is the notion that people can continuously improve their work. By continuously examining processes and outcomes, people can make their work more effective. Quality improvement contends that most things can be improved, and such improvement builds upon traditional quality assurance methods by emphasizing process improvements at an organization and system level. The principles of CQI build upon the concept that an iterative process of change for improvement depends upon student involvement for detecting which changes should be made (Boer, Berger, Chapman, & Gertsen, 2000). CQI process starts with a clear understanding of mission, constituencies, and objectives of a higher-education institute. The establishment of cooperative and collaborative practice aims at quality improvement. CQI principles have helped to improve outcomes for customers, customer satisfaction, workforce retention and satisfaction, use of prevention interventions, best practices and innovation, waste reduction, rework reduction, error reduction, cost effectiveness, and processes of services (e.g., responsiveness, availability, timeliness, cultural sensitivity, effectiveness, and efficiency). At the core of CQI, a simple question is asked, "*how can we do better?*" CQI defines quality as meeting and/or exceeding expectations. As a majority of problems are commonly found in processes, CQI focuses on "process" improvement rather than on the individual. Unintended variation in processes can lead to unwanted variations in outcomes. As such, CQI seeks to reduce or eliminate unwanted variations. CQI is most effective when it becomes a natural part of the way everyday work is done or where a culture of embracing CQI is evident.

CQI principles are based on the concepts of planned, organized, systematic, ongoing, and incremental change of existing practices aimed at improving overall performance (Boer et al., 2000). To operationalize CQI, Sonpal-Valias (2009) identified a CQI cycle as the following of "Plan - Do - Check - Reflect - Act":

- *Plan* programs and services
- *Deliver* them
- *Measure* performance
- *Interpret* performance and identify ways to improve it
- *Choose and implement* strategies to improve our systems and processes
- Start a new cycle again

CONTINUOUS QUALITY IMPROVEMENT: ACCREDITATION

In nursing, accreditation criteria are developed using the principles of quality improvement. The timeframe (e.g., 5 to 10 years) used in nursing accreditation reflects a quality circle to examine or review if defined objectives and specificities are met. The philosophical underpinning of nursing accreditation is that maintaining quality is essential. Accreditation is a peer-reviewed and voluntary process in which the school or the program asks for an external review of its educational programs, facilities, student learning and outcomes, and faculty. The U.S. Department of Education recognizes two accreditation agencies for nursing: The Commission on Collegiate Nursing Education (CCNE) and the National League for Nursing Accrediting Commission (NLNAC). In addition, all baccalaureate nursing programs must be approved by the State Board of Nursing so that their graduates can sit for the licensing examinations offered by the National Council of States of Boards of Nursing, Inc. The State Board of Nursing uses benchmarks (e.g., NCLEX pass rates, admission criteria, clinical sites, qualification of nurse educators) to evaluate nursing programs. An annual report to the State Board of Nursing is often required, which serves a purpose for formative evaluations of the nursing program.

Accreditation in nursing is considered on two levels—the accreditation of the university or college and the accreditation of the nursing program (Amos, 2005). Peers comprised of experienced educators in nursing education conduct accreditation reviews of a respective program to assess program quality and integrity according to the established standards. CCNE, for example, set four standards for evaluating nursing program quality, including Standard I: Mission and governance; Standard II: Instructional commitment and resources; Standard III: Curriculum and teaching learning practices, and Standard IV: Program effectiveness: Aggregate student and faculty outcomes (2009). The NLNAC (2008) has issued six standards and they are mission and administrative capacity, faculty and staff, students, curriculum, resources, and outcomes.

Accreditation applies CQI principles in which faculty and administrators conduct self-evaluation prior to the accreditation's site visit. The self-evaluation is based on standards established by CCNE or the NLNAC (as noted earlier). The self-evaluation process engages faculty and administrators through their examination of mission and governance, curriculum, academic policies, assessment of learning, student and faculty achievements, educational resources, and identification of strengths and weaknesses or areas for improvement. In the self-evaluation process, each standard is assessed to see if there is any compliance issue, a gap, and/or weakness area needing improvement; if so, recommendations are made and ways for quality improvement are described, and efforts are made on sustaining and improving the quality and integrity of the nursing program. The cycle of accreditation, ranging from 5 years to a maximum 10 years, provides a regular interval for examining quality and integrity of a nursing program, and ultimately, striving for excellence of nursing education.

CONTINUOUS QUALITY IMPROVEMENT: ACHIEVING EXCELLENCE

Quality is everyone's business and excellence is its goal. The National League for Nursing (NLN, 2011) has recently defined CQI in this light as well: engagement in a variety of activities that promote excellence. Here, excellence is defined as "superiority, first class, great merit or efficiency" (Merriam-Webster, 2011). In 2006, the NLN previously unveiled the *Excellence in Nursing Education Model* at its educational summit, which comprises eight core elements:

- A well-prepared faculty
- Student-centered, interactive, and innovative programs and curricula
- Evidence-based programs and teaching/evaluation methods
- Qualified students
- Clear program standards and hallmarks that raise expectations
- Means to recognize expertise
- Quality and adequate resources
- Well-prepared educational administrators

The NLN's Excellence in Nursing Education Model outlines hallmarks, indicators, glossaries, and references. Hallmarks of excellence are thought of as characteristics or traits that serve to define a level of outstanding performance (2011). Quality improvement to achieve excellence focuses on broad areas, including students, faculty, curriculum, teaching/learning/evaluation strategies, resources, innovation, educational research, environment, and leadership. Major constituencies are also considered and they may include students and their families, faculty, staff, administrators, institution, community key players, and the public. CQI helps improve processes toward excellence as it allows evaluation of internal processes and external outcomes of accelerated nursing programs on an ongoing basis. The following highlights three major areas—students, faculty, and curriculum—using CQI to achieve excellence in accelerated nursing education.

Accelerated Students

Students' learning and learning outcomes are key quality indicators. Of course, most students enrolled in accelerated nursing programs are second-degree students. And although the profile of accelerated students is yet to be well documented, research has begun to describe these students as "chronologically older," "mature," "motivated," "self-directed," and having more life experiences and higher expectations for educational processes and outcomes than those of traditional students (AACN, 2005; Miklancie & Davis, 2005; Raines & Spies, 2007; Roberts et al., 2001.). Other studies found that accelerated students were not afraid to challenge instructors and had the right balance between intellectual ability and emotional fortitude. Accelerated students may view education and faculty more critically. Those with a college degree in business use a business-related style and focus on a goal that helps result in their job advancement (Bradshaw & Nugent, 1997; Quellet, MacIntosh, Gibson, & Jefferson, 2008; Rouse & Rooda, 2010). Anecdotally, some faculty members have described accelerated students as "assertive," "challenging," "critical," and sometimes "demanding."

Studies found that attrition rates tended to be higher in accelerated nursing programs than in traditional BSN programs (Bentley, 2006; Seldomridge & DiBartolo, 2005). Stress is identified as one of the contributing factors to attrition since the accelerated program accomplishes programmatic objectives in a short time, with the assumption that students can build on previous learning experiences. Instruction, which has its own intensity with courses offered full-time and no breaks between sessions, often uses a frontloaded didactic instruction and immersed clinical practicum. Students receive the same number of clinical hours and content areas as their counterparts in traditional entry-level nursing programs. The workload, intensity, rigor, time demands, and personal stress commonly challenge students in accelerated programs (Meyer, Hoover, & Maposa, 2006). It is also challenging for accelerated students to incorporate professional formation and role development values in such a condensed timeframe (Speziale, 2002). Although the admission standard for accelerated students is typically high (minimum 3.0 GPA), failure to identify individuals who have already proven their ability to succeed at a college or university may also contribute to the high attrition rates. Anecdotally, other factors may contribute to the attrition, such as a lack of rigorous academic support services, suboptimal quality in teaching (both didactic and clinical due to novice educators), and/or a less promising job market in the students' areas (White, Wax, & Berrey, 2000; Yearwood, Singleton, Feldman, & Colombraro, 2001; Zhan, 2009).

The mission of accelerated nursing education is to provide high quality education for preparation of nursing graduates to meet the ever-changing health care needs. To this end, quality indicators for assessment and improvement require students to exhibit a "spirit of inquiry" while committing to lifelong learning, innovation, continuous quality performance improvement, and a career in nursing (NLN, 2011). What strategies can be used to address challenges and promote success for accelerated students? A CQI method helps focus on process improvement directed toward achieving excellence in students' learning and faculty teaching.

CQI requires clearly defined learning outcomes (quality). Measurable tools or methods are needed for data collection. Formative and summative assessments are also needed, implying something we do "*with*" and "*for*" students, while both types of assessments share a common goal of evaluating student knowledge. The key distinction between the formative and summative assessments is the purpose for which the evaluation is implemented. Formative assessment informs and guides adjustments in the process of teaching/learning, whereas summative evaluation monitors progress and overall success on a long-term basis. In formative assessment, faculty provide feedback to students when faculty recognize student learning gaps and close those gaps. Using quizzes and tests on a weekly or biweekly basis affords an opportunity for identifying learning gaps while students are learning. The "Minute paper" is another way to not only collect students' feedback on teaching but also to enable students to reflect on their own learning. Reviewing exams helps students identify strengths and weaknesses in learning. Greater attention is given to providing advice for students' improvement, and thus improving quality of their learning.

Summative assessment occurs at the end of each course, semester, and program in the form of comprehensive examinations and capstone projects. Students shared learning goals and objectives at the very beginning of courses and are involved in self-assessments during the course of their learning. Adequate academic support services tailored to meeting students' learning needs are provided. Students' leadership development, such as participating in a nursing student organization, is strongly encouraged and supported. Student satisfaction is a critical indicator for program quality, and should also assess what resources are needed, when resources are needed, accessibility of resources, and faculty availability to students. Students have unique learning styles that require varied teaching approaches and resources. It is not enough to use student performance as the only indicator of quality; evaluation of student satisfaction is critical as well.

Both formative and summative evaluations provide data necessary for recommending actions for quality improvement. Unlike a traditional view that seeks equal quality of learning outcomes, the CQI approach brings focus on outcomes and moves from microassessment in the classroom to macroassessment of the program. CQI also helps process improvement by adjustment of teaching pedagogy in concert with students' feedback, while also considering students' learning needs and styles. Overall program improvement occurs through recommendations for the next cycle of CQI, always aimed at ensuring success of accelerated nursing students.

Faculty

Accelerated education in nursing is a new territory to many faculty and sometimes even to seasoned educators. Quality of the nursing program requires a faculty complement that includes a cadre of individuals who not only have expertise and experience as educators and clinicians, but also embrace the institution's mission and goals. The severe shortage of doctorally prepared faculty in nursing makes having a cadre of qualified nurse educators quite challenging, and thus deliberately searching for and retaining faculty with excellence in education, clinical practice, and/or research is an ongoing effort. Strategies are needed to retain qualified nursing faculty who are critical for quality and integrity of the accelerated nursing program.

An assessment is needed to identify knowledge and skill gaps of faculty for their teaching in an accelerated program, as some faculty may not be familiar with teaching accelerated curriculum and students. Ongoing support for faculty teaching in the accelerated nursing program may involve faculty development activities based on an individual goal plan, a mentoring program, teambuilding and teaching, and a train the trainers approach. Faculty members require clear communication about their roles, expectations, accountability, and responsibility in academia. To promote excellence in faculty's area of expertise, faculty members are encouraged to be involved in quality improvement activities aimed toward achieving excellence in their teaching, service, and research, the three broadly defined areas for assessing faculty performance in academia.

Most nursing students in accelerated programs are highly motivated and self-directed, and thus, flexible and creative methods of teaching are encouraged. Teaching strategies may include recognizing students' prior college experiences and incorporating higher levels of cognitive and affective information into the course objectives (Cangelosi, 2007). Based on assessment data, an in-depth orientation to the role of faculty is designed and implemented. A mentoring program to assist faculty as they progress in their career is imperative and anecdotally this approach helps retain nurse educators. An established set of faculty competencies is used to prepare individuals for the faculty role and to help faculty maintain competence/expertise in their roles (NLN, 2011). Adequate planning, timely communication, fair and comprehensive performance review, and a quality improvement focus create a less stressful environment for faculty.

Teaching effectiveness is assessed by students' evaluations and peer evaluations in some institutions. Each faculty has the responsibility to continue to improve and implement course changes that benefit the students and encourage the accomplishment of course objectives. Using a CQI approach, an ongoing evaluation of teaching is implemented as faculty may miss an important learning opportunity if the end-of-course evaluations are the only input received from students regarding the course quality (Watt, Simpson, McKillop, & Nunn, 2002). By encouraging anonymous and frequent evaluative dialogue between faculty and students, a continuous improvement cycle is established. If it is used properly, such dialogue may allow the faculty to improve courses more effectively (Ballantyne, 1999) and students may feel empowered in their learning, as their feedback matters in the process of learning.

CQI promotes using data to analyze and improve processes (Dickerson, 2000). In teaching, CQI involves focusing on students' learning and outcomes of their learning. "Minute papers" are used as a means to get formative feedback from students in the teaching process. The use of minute papers has been an effective way of eliciting constructive feedback during the course of a class and of evaluating the accomplishment of course objectives (Stead, 2005). This technique allows students one minute at the end of class to let the faculty know what they learned and any problems they may have had with the class. In addition to minute papers, the evidence shows that midcourse evaluations also demonstrate a correlation between their use and the improvement of final course evaluations. If students are not asked for feedback until the end-of-course student evaluations, feedback needed to improve the course might not be timely enough for improving faculty teaching and student learning (Vits & Gelders, 2002). By increasing the frequency of student feedback, faculty may alter the iterative cycle of change and facilitate continuous as well as expeditious course improvement (Middel, Boer, & Fisscher, 2006). Formative evaluations (e.g., minute papers, midcourse evaluations, online surveys, and e-mails) provide faculty with students' feedback that helps faculty see what works and what needs to be improved. The Association of American Colleges and Universities (2004) views student achievement of intended learning outcomes as the key indicator of collegiate quality and has its motto, "*We have not taught if our students have not learned.*"

Curriculum

A curriculum is a set of courses and their contents used to plan and guide students' learning. Since accelerated nursing programs are designed in a condensed time frame, the curriculum is designed to be innovative to ensure that students are well prepared for competently entering the nursing profession and/or assume a leadership role in health care settings. As nursing education prepares lifelong learners, the accelerated curriculum focuses on what students "*must know*" rather than what would be "*nice to know*" due to the short timeframe of the program of study.

Knowledge is evolving, so are essential competencies and requirements from accrediting agencies, State Boards of Nursing, Institute of Medicine, and the public. AACN, for example, revised its essentials of baccalaureate (BSN) education for professional nursing practice in 2008 and its essentials for master's education in nursing (MSN) in 2011. The BSN essentials include liberal education for baccalaureate generalist nursing practice, basic organizational and system leadership for quality care and patient safety, scholarship for evidence-based practice, information management and application of patient care technology, health care policy, finance, and regulatory environments, interprofessional communication and collaboration for improving patient health outcomes, clinical prevention and population health, professionalism and professional values, and baccalaureate generalist nursing practice.

The MSN essentials include background for practice from sciences and humanities, organizational and system leadership, quality improvement and safety, translating and integrating scholarship into practice, informatics and health care technologies, health policy and advocacy, interprofessional collaboration for improving patient and population health outcomes, clinical prevention and population health for improving health, and master's-level nursing practice. Accelerated curriculum, therefore, is based on concepts and frameworks that reflect new essentials and core competencies, such as evidence-based practice, professional formation, technology infusion, quality improvement and safety, and leadership development. Example courses or contents are *nursing informatics, genetics and genomics in nursing and health, safety and quality*, and *gerontological nursing.*

NLN (2011) outlines benchmarks for assessing curriculum using the principle of CQI. CQI is a comprehensive, sustained, and integrative approach to systematic curriculum assessment to examine whether the curriculum (a) is flexible and current and allows regular refinement to incorporate current societal and health care trends and issues, research findings, innovative practices, and local as well as global perspectives; (b) provides experiential cultural learning activities that promote students' thinking abilities; (c) emphasizes professional formation that promotes lifelong learning, values development, and creativity; (d) develops leadership roles that prepare graduates to improve quality, safety, and outcomes of patient and health care; and (e) supports evidence-based practice.

In nursing education, the curriculum committee comprised of faculty uses the CQI approach to regularly review, refine, and redesign the nursing curriculum. Successful practice includes carefully planned curriculum, committee designated for curricular review and refinement, and ongoing dialogs among faculty about curriculum with respect to new essentials, competencies, and evolving knowledge and technologies. Curriculum mapping may be used as it is a collaborative and reflective process that helps teaching and learning, and enables the faculty to assure that essentials are integrated into the curriculum.

CONTINUOUS QUALITY IMPROVEMENT: LEADERSHIP

A Culture of Quality Improvement

Creation of a culture that embraces quality and its improvement requires strong leadership at all levels to articulate a vision and inspire a lasting commitment to achieve high quality and integrity of accelerated nursing programs. Continuous quality improvement is a constant, gradual, and incremental approach to improve quality. Educational leaders commit to creating an environment and culture where quality and its improvement are valued and embraced by all involved. Further, an organization culture of values, beliefs, and norms shapes human behaviors. Assessment of organizational culture helps implement CQI. Critical questions are asked: *"What are values and norms associated with teamwork?", "Are risk-taking and innovation valued?"*, and *"What are norms and values associated in hierarchical levels?"*

To bring about changes in the higher-education setting, leaders must be intentional and reflective, conscientiously pursue change strategies, and work within norms and structures of the academy (Brown & Marshall, 2008). Numerous tools (flow charts, histograms, benchmarking, fishbone diagrams, decision trees or matrices, nominal group technique, consensus building) can be used to identify and prioritize program problems and projects. Collectively, a number of these elements are referred to as the CQI tool kit (Dew & Nearing, 2004). This commitment helps create an environment and culture in higher education in which everyone takes ownership of improved education and where high value is placed on communication, collaboration, and teamwork. The goal is to achieve high quality and integrity of educational programs.

Teambuilding

Faculty and staff teamwork and team decision making are necessary for quality improvements. Teambuilding requires construction of the team that eventually shares a common understanding of systems and processes for quality improvement. Basic elements of team construction may include goals and specific outcomes. The leader establishes the linkages between strategic goals and team functional activities aimed toward quality improvement. Team success lies in the fundamental conditions that allow effective task processes to emerge and cause members to engage in these processes. Three conditions for teambuilding include (1) trust among members, (2) a sense of group identity, and (3) a sense of group efficacy. These conditions are essential to team effectiveness (Druskat & Wolff, 2001; Porter-O'Grady & Malloch, 2007).

Teams are small systems. CQI needs to be built on the principles at the team system level, including (1) a focus on process improvement; (2) an information/data-based decision making approach; (3) teamwork; (4) a link between CQI and strategic goals; (5) assessment of goals for improvement; and (6) flexibility in implementing quality improvement approaches. The amount of time that needs to be spent on teambuilding or process improvement is much more effective than a managers-involved-only approach (Porter-O'Grady & Malloch, 2007). Critical to faculty/staff participation is education and training, empowerment, open communication, and recognition. Support for faculty and staff is needed for quality improvement work and for taking ownership of improved education. High value is placed on commitment to communication, collaboration, and teamwork as CQI involves small steps, a group effort, a focus on processes, and people who understand and commit to quality standards.

Strategic Planning

A CQI process begins with a clear understanding of what one is trying to achieve. A strategic plan provides a clear aim and helps establish priorities as to specific objectives to be accomplished in a timeframe. The strategic plan serves as a roadmap toward goals and objectives. Strategic planning is a process that involves faculty, staff, and students in setting goals for the respective accelerated nursing program. In the planning process, choices are made as to what to do and what not to do through analysis of strength, weakness, threats, and opportunities. Needed resources are identified and analyzed. Indicators/benchmarks and valid measurements are identified and used. In the strategic planning process, fundamental questions are asked: *Where are we now? (Assessment) Where do we need to be? (Gap/Future End State) How will we close the gap? (Strategic Plan) How will we monitor the progress? (CQI)* A good strategic plan balances between what the nursing program/school/college is capable of doing versus what the nursing program/school/college would like to do and covers a sufficient time period to close the performance gap. Decisions are guided at the level of nursing faculty, staff, students, and community major stakeholders.

Strategic planning in accelerated programs is a process inclusive of faculty and community key players. It is knowledge based, process oriented, and quality targeted. The CQI cycle (depicted below) shows the integration of a strategic plan along with purposeful data collection, evaluation (interpretation of facts), and action (feedback to support decision making and improve processes).

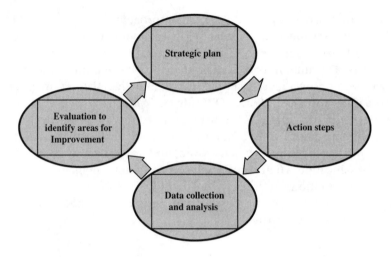

Data-Driven Decision Making

CQI is built on the principle of information/data-based decision making. It involves managing by facts by asking *"What is the problem?"*, *"What are facts/data?,"* and *"What are decisions to bring resolves?"* Data-driven decision making can be aided by process mapping, flowcharts, focused group interviews, online surveys, and/or participatory observations. Measuring the problem and bringing resolution are both part of managing by factual analysis. In essence, CQI evaluations are used to assess the effectiveness of an action step/process/activity, give direction for improvement, and create a cycle of feedback and improvement within the process itself. A CQI approach involves measuring short-term outcomes at the action level and the outcome of each objective. The established evaluation plan helps capture critical data elements. Leading indicators for measurement in accelerated nursing education are based on accreditation standards and criteria, as noted earlier. At least one target for each measurement is recommended. The merit of using targeted measure is intended to put focus on one's strategy. As each target is reached, strategy is successfully executed. To plan, collect, and use data facilitate effective decision making, and allow testing and refining changes necessary for quality improvement.

A Healthy Workplace

Workers spend at least one-third of their lifetime in workplace before retirement. A healthy academic environment is an important indicator of quality and integrity in accelerated nursing programs.

World Health Organization (WHO, 2010) defines a healthy workplace as follows:

> A healthy workplace is a place where everyone works together to achieve an agreed vision for the health and well-being of workers and the surrounding community. It provides all members of the workforce with physical, psychological, social and organizational conditions that protect and promote health and safety. It enables managers and workers to increase control over their own health and to improve it, and to become more energetic, positive and contented. (p. 15).

The WHO calls for a collaborative commitment to promote healthy work environments that support and foster excellence and humanity. National organizations in nursing have advocated for promoting healthy work environments that are important for safety and quality of patient care, for retention of nursing staff and faculty, and for excellence in nursing education (American Association of Critical-Care Nurses, 2005; American Organization of Nurse Executives, 2004; National League for Nursing, 2006). National League for Nursing (2006) has published the *Healthy Work Environment Tool Kit* that addresses nine work-related areas: salaries, benefits, workload, collegial environment, role preparation and professional development, scholarship, institutional support, marketing and recognition, and leadership. The American Association of Critical-Care Nurses (2005) has initiated the dialog among clinical nurses regarding a healthy workplace and its impact on quality of patient care and quality of nurses' work life. The American Association of Critical-Care Nurses has established six standards for building and sustaining a healthy workplace, namely skilled communication, true collaboration, effective decision making, appropriate staffing, meaningful recognition, and authentic leadership.

The phenomenon of work environments is multifaceted. Mounting evidence shows that unhealthy work environments, namely bully, sabotage, negativity, divisiveness, disrespectfulness, deceptiveness, and harassment, contribute to ineffectiveness, errors, conflicts, stress, demoralization, psychological trauma, and unsafe. Academic mobbing, a form of engaged and pathological behaviors of humiliation and unjustified accusation toward a target(s), is a threat to workplace health and safety, an ugly phenomenon that affects about 20 million U.S. workers (Rushton, 2006). Academic leaders must be able to recognize an early sign of mobbing and resolve the conflict before it escalates, as leadership is needed to influence and determine the culture of the organization and the overall health of the academic setting. Building, sustaining, and promoting healthy work environments require academic leaders' commitment to translate core values—caring, integrity, diversity, transparency, truthfulness, and honesty—into daily practice. To lead the way, these values are shared and communicated among faculty, staff, and students. Necessary steps shall be taken to remove negativity and divisiveness so that collegiality is supported and a healthy work environment can be maintained.

Transformation

Implementing CQI needs transformational leadership. The leader must communicate a clear vision of why quality improvement is necessary and seek buy-in from all involved. Status quo is challenged. Creativity is encouraged among faculty, staff, and students, while encouraging new ways of doing things and new opportunities to learn. Lines of communication are open so that people feel free to share ideas in the process of improvement. To engage, empower, and enable others to implement quality improvement requires leaders to let go of responsibilities that others can perform, and focus upon encouragement of initiatives, ideas, and risk taking. The leader must also ensure that people have goals and receive feedback on their performance. The leader develops, empowers, coaches to ensure success, and reinforces good work and good attempts, while also sharing information, knowledge, skills, and values. The leader trusts and respects each individual while providing support without taking over (Lolly, 1996).

FUTURE DIRECTIONS: CHALLENGES AND STRATEGIES

American Society for Quality (ASQ) is a global community of experts and the leading authority on quality. ASQ has a vision for making quality a global priority, an organizational imperative, and a personal ethic. Higher education is urged to shift its focus from one in quantitative expansion to one with an emphasis on quality (Sahney, Banwet, & Karunes, 2004). Academe has an increased interest in adopting CQI as higher education has become complex and competitive. Application of CQI to manage and improve the quality of higher education—students, faculty, programs, resources, and environment—is essential. Successful implementation of CQI in academe demands transformative leadership and a culture change in which faculty, staff, students, and administrators need to buy in and commit to it. A cultural change is challenging and involves deconstructing habitual thinking and behaviors so that open-ended and ongoing quality improvement is embraced and practiced. Leaders must have commitment to create an environment and organizational culture for continuous quality improvement for all involved in higher education.

CQI is essential in particular for accelerated education since its curriculum delivery is condensed in a short timeframe and often requires innovation. CQI provides a process-oriented and teamwork-spirited approach to ensure high quality and integrity of nursing education. Leadership commitment, inclusion of faculty, students, and staff, valid measurements, data/information-based decision making, and gaps analysis help continue improvement of the accelerated nursing programs. Implementing CQI is challenging since its effectiveness can not only come from the management team; instead, CQI comes from all involved in the nursing program. Strategies can be used to implement CQI, including Mission and Values reflective of a quality culture. Leadership at all levels are required to commit to CQI to sustain the efforts of CQI, use CQI as a means to develop an organization into a fully integrated system, engage faculty in designing and implementing CQI, articulate and communicate CQI methods and steps, conduct critical analysis for processes to be improved, plan change and development or training accordingly, and evaluate and formulate a plan for the next identified process for improvement. The commitment to quality is a must in higher education. CQI, when embedded in an organizational culture, will not only enhance accelerated nursing programs but will also benefit the public and society as a whole.

REFERENCES

American Association of Colleges of Nursing. (2005). *AACN Issue Bulletin: Accelerated programs: The fast-track to careers in nursing.* Retrieved May 2011 from http://www.aacn.nche.edu/publications/issues/Aug02.htm

American Association of Colleges of Nursing. (2010). *Fact sheet: Accelerated baccalaureate and master's degrees in nursing.* Retrieved January 2011 from http://www.aacn.nche.edu/media/factsheets/acceleratedprog.htm

American Association of Critical-Care Nurse. (2005). *AACN standards for establishing and sustaining healthy work environment.* Retrieved June 20, 2011 from www.aacn.org/WD/HWE/Docs/HWEStandards.pdf

American Organization of Nurse Executives (2004). *Principles and elements of a healthful practice/work environment.* Retrieved June 15, 2011 from http://www.aone.org/aone/pdf/Principlesandelementshealthfulworkpractice.pdf

American Society for Quality. (2011). *Common quality issues in education [online].* Retrieved March 25 from http://www.asq.org/education/why-quality/common-issues.html

Amos, L. (2005). *Baccalaureate nursing programs.* Retrieved April 5, 2011 from www.aacn.nech.edu/nurse_ed/BSNArticle.htm

Association of American College and Universities (2004). *Taking responsibility for the quality of the baccalaureate degree*. Washington, DC: Author.

Ballantyne, C. (1999). Improving university teaching: Responding to feedback from students. *In* N. Zepke, M. Knight, L Leach, & A Viskovic (Eds). *Adult learning culture: Challenges and choices in times of change*. p. 155–165. WP Press, Wellington.

Bentley, R. (2006, May/June). Comparison of traditional and accelerated baccalaureate nursing graduates. *Nurse Educator, 31*(2), 79–83.

Boer, H., Berger, A., Chapman, R., & Gertsen, F. (2000). *CI changes: From suggestion box to organizational learning: Continuous improvement in Europe and Australia*. Aldershot, UK: Ashgate.

Bradshaw, M. J., & Nugent, K. (1997). Clinical learning experiences of non-traditional age nursing students [News, Notes, & Tips]. *Nurse Educator, 22*(6), 40–47.

Brown, J. F., & Marshall, B. L (2008). Continuous quality improvement: An effective strategy for improving of program outcomes in a higher education setting. *Nursing Education Perspectives, 29*(4), 205–211.

Business Dictionary. (2011). Retrieved June 20, 2011 from www.businessdictionary.com/defintiion/quality-improvement.html

Cangelosi, P. R. (2007). Voices of graduates from second-degree baccalaureate nursing programs. *Journal of Professional Nursing, 23*(2), 91–97.

Carroll, D. P. (1992). *Notes on nursing by Florence Nightingale*. J. B. Lippincott Company, PA.

Commission on Collegiate Nursing Education. (2009). Standards for accreditation of baccalaureate and graduate nursing programs. Retrieved June 1, 2011 from www.aacn.nche.edu/accreditation

Deming, W. E. (1986). *Out of the crisis*. Massachusetts Institute of Technology, Center for Advanced Engineering Study, Cambridge, MA.

Dew, J. R., & Nearing, M. M. (2004). *Continuous quality improvement in higher education*. Westport, CT: Praeger.

Dickerson, P. S. (2000). A CQI approach to evaluating continuing education: Processes and outcomes. *Journal for Nurses in Staff Development, 16*, 34–40.

Donabedian, A. (1989). The end results of health care. Ernest Codman's contribution to quality assessment and beyond. *The Millbank Quarterly, 67*(2), 233–234.

Downey, T. S. (2000). The application of continuous quality improvement models in methods to higher education: Can we learn from business? In *Cross-Roads of the New Millennium Proceedings of the Technological Education and National Development conference* (p. 10), April 8–10, Abu Dhabi, United Arab Emirates.

Druskat, V. U., & Wolff, S. B. (2001). Building the emotional intelligence of groups. *Harvard Business Review, 79*(3), 81–90.

Lolly, E. (1996). Transformative leadership, a presentation given at the 1996 Ohio Literacy Resource Center Leadership Institute, OH.

Merriam-Webster. (2011). Retrieved March 28, 2011 from www.marriam-webster.com/dictionary/excellent

Meyer, G. A., Hoover, K. G., & Maposa, S. (2006, August). A profile of accelerated BSN graduates (2004). *Journal of Nursing Education, 45*(8), 324–327.

Middel, R., Boer, H., & Fisscher, O. (2006). Continuous improvement and collaborative improvement: Similarities and differences. *Creativity and Innovation Management, 15*(4), 338–347.

Miklancie, M., & Davis, T. (2005). The second-degree accelerated program as an innovative educational strategy: New century, new chapter, new challenge. *Nursing Education Perspectives, 26*(5), 291–294.

National League for Nursing. (2006). *The healthy work environment tool kit.* Retrieved June 20, 2011 from http://www.nln.org/facultydevelopment/healthy-workenvironment/toolkit.pdf

National League for Nursing. (2011). Retrieved May 6, 2011 from www.nln.org/excellence/hallmarks_indicators.htm

National League for Nursing Accreditation Commission. (2008). NLNAC Standards and Criteria Baccalaureate. Retrieved May 20, 2011 from www.nlnac.org/manuals/SC2008_baccalaureate.pdf

Porter-O'Grady, T., & Malloch, K. (2007). *Quantum leadership: A resource for health care innovation* (2nd ed.). Sudbury, MA: Jones & Bartlett Publishers.

Quellet, L. L., MacIntosh, J., Gibson, C. H., & Jefferson, S. (2008, February). Evaluation of selected outcomes of an accelerated nursing degree program. *Nursing Education Today, 28*(2), 194–201.

Raines, D. A., & Spies, A. (2007, November/December). One year later: Reflections and work activities of accelerated second-degree Bachelor of Science in Nursing Graduates. *Journal of Professional Nursing, 23*(6), 329–334.

Roberts, K., Mason, J., & Wood, P. (2001, December). A comparison of a traditional and an accelerated basic nursing education program. *Contemporary Nurse, 11*(2/3), 283–287.

Rouse, S. M., & Rooda, L. A. (2010, June 1). Factors for attrition in an accelerated baccalaureate nursing program. *Journal of Nursing Education, 49*(6), 359–362.

Rushton, P. (2006). Academic mobbing. Retrieved on June 28, 2011 from http://academicmobbing.blogspot.com/

Sahney, S., Banwet, D. K., & Karunes, S. (2004). Conceptualizing total quality management in higher education. *The TQM Magazine, 16*(2), 145–159.

Seldomridge, L. A., & DiBartolo, M. C. (2005, March-April). A profile of accelerated second bachelor's degree nursing students. *Nurse Educator, 30*(2), 65–68.

Sonpal-Valias, N. (2009). *Outcome evaluation: Definition and overview.* Calgary, AB, Canada: The Vocational and Rehabilitation Research Institute.

Speziale, H. (2002). RN-MSN admission practices and curricular in the mid-Atlantic region. *Nursing Education Perspectives, 23*(6), 294–299.

Stead, D. (2005). A review of the one-minute paper. *Active Learning in Higher Education, 6*(2), 118–131.

Steyn, G. (2000). Applying principles of total quality management to a learning process: A case study. *South African Journal of Higher Education, 14*(1), 174–184.

Ulrich, B. T. (1992). *Leadership and management according to Florence Nightingale* (pp. 2–6, 10–58). Norwalk: Appleton & Kange,

Vits, J., & Gelders, L. (2002). Performance improvement theory. *International Journal of Production Economics, 77*(3), 285–298.

Vora, M. (2002). Business excellence through quality management. *Total Quality Management & Business Excellence, 13*(8), 1151–1159.

Walton, M. (1988). *The Deming management method*. New York, NY: The Berkley Publishing Group.

Watt, S., Simpson, C., McKillop, C., & Nunn, V. (2002). Electronic course surveys: Does automating feedback and reporting give better results? *Assessment and Evaluation in Higher Education, 27*(4), 325–337.

White, K., Wax, W., & Berrey, A. (2000, September-October). Accelerated second degree advanced practice nurses: How do they fare in the job market? *Nursing Outlook, 48*(5), 218–222.

World Health Organization. (2010). *WHO healthy workplace framework and model: Background document and supporting literature and practices*. Retrieved June 20 2011 from http://www.who.inf/occupational_health/healthy_workplace_framework_pdf

Yearwood, E., Singleton, J., Feldman, H., & Colombraro, G. (2001). A case study in implementing CQI in a nursing education program. *Journal of Professional Nursing, 17*, 297–304.

Zhan, L. (2009). Personal communication with accelerated BSN students, May 20, Boston, MA.

Chapter 9

Current and Future Needs of Accelerated Nursing Programs: Faculty Recruitment, Retention, and Development

Kathy Rideout

S uccessful academic programs are characterized by a triad of rigorous curriculum, exceptional students, and stellar, highly committed faculty. Recruitment and retention of excellent faculty to teach in an accelerated nursing program and their ongoing development is critical to ensure continued success of these programs. The challenges, strategies, and future directions for each of these issues will be discussed in this chapter.

FACULTY RECRUITMENT

Challenges

With the nursing faculty shortage upon us, it is essential that we develop mechanisms to successfully recruit the best and the brightest individuals to become faculty. During the academic year 2005–2006, the National League for Nursing (NLN) and the Carnegie Foundation Preparation for the Professions Program conducted a study involving nurse educators. This study, involving approximately 32,000 nurse educators, highlighted three main contributing factors to the nursing faculty shortage: aging faculty, increased workload, and inadequate financial compensation (Kaufman, 2007). Findings from the 2009 NLN Faculty Census noted that full-time nursing educators over the age of 60 increased from 9% in

2006 to nearly 16% in 2009 and that "fifty-seven percent of part-time educators and nearly 76 percent of full-time faculty were over the age of 45 in 2009" (Kaufman, 2009, p. 1).

Ensuring that faculty who are teaching in an accelerated program are clinically competent and current in their clinical practice is crucial. Nurses graduating from PhD programs may not have current clinical competence, focusing mainly on research initiatives. This fact further limits the number of PhD-prepared faculty who can provide clinical supervision in an accelerated program.

Just as important, and more challenging at times, is to ensure that someone who is clinically competent can also teach. Sweitzer (2003) notes that it is critical to remember that just because someone is a skilled practitioner does not guarantee that the person will be a good educator. The challenge is to develop strategies that are of high quality, cost effective, and efficient while assisting/preparing the excellent clinician to become an excellent educator/teacher. Preparing students to be our future nurses is a skill unto itself and selected competencies need to be acquired to ensure a quality of graduates and educational program. Becoming a faculty member will require learning the new skill set that is much different than that of a clinician and the new learning required may be exciting for some but a barrier to others.

The salaries for faculty may also be a disincentive. Therefore, helping to find a way by which their income will not be negatively affected by becoming a faculty member is another challenge. Kaufman (2009) noted in the 2009 NLN Faculty Census Data that nursing faculty earn significantly less that other faculty across higher education; professors in nursing earn 45% less than comparatively ranked non-nurse faculty, while associate and assistant professors earn 19% and 15% less, respectively. In *The Nursing Faculty Shortage: A Crisis for Health Care* (Yordy, 2006), public institutions are less competitive in relation to salaries, as they are constrained by state and local budgets that are "burdened by reduced federal funds, increasing Medicaid costs, crumbling infractures, and pressures to shore up public school systems" (p. 4). This report further notes that as health care organizations increase nursing salaries to meet the demands of the nursing shortage, the gap between clinicians and faculty salaries will worsen (Yordy, 2006).

Ensuring that the educational preparation required and preferred for a faculty member (minimally master's prepared for clinical instruction and doctorally prepared for didactic instruction) is achieved during the recruitment process can also be a significant challenge. Frequently, a nurse who is interested in teaching may not have the preferred educational preparation and therefore unable to pursue a career in teaching.

Despite these challenges, several strategies can be implemented to assist in the recruitment of excellent faculty.

Strategies

It is easier to recruit faculty to teach in an accelerated program that is renowned for excellence, and therefore, it is critical to ensure that the curriculum is solid and its graduates are competent and exemplary. Strategic marketing of the program should reflect the successful outcomes of its graduates and the satisfaction of the faculty teaching in the program. Creative uses of the school's webpage can highlight the school's successes and its graduates' achievements. This positive attention to the program will attract new faculty who want to be a part of a successful enterprise.

Potential faculty recruits must be willing and interested to learn a faculty role, and to be competent in their nursing skills. Educational offerings from seasoned faculty could be provided to educate novice faculty in the role, responsibilities, and expectations of teaching. Flexibility on the part of nursing school administration is key to maintain a balance of clinical and teaching expertise. Allowing nursing faculty the opportunity to blend their teaching role with a clinical practice role could further enhance the attraction of assuming a faculty position.

An outstanding source for recruiting potential faculty may come from collaborative affiliations with clinical agencies. Nurses who are prepared as clinical nurse specialists or nurse practitioners already possess the advance clinical skills necessary to teach in an undergraduate program. Depending on the nurses' current practice site and the agency's clinical needs, it may be possible to arrange for joint appointments between the clinical agency and the school of nursing. Mathews (2003) noted that it is time to bring "educators from clinical and academic settings together to share experiences, knowledge, and skills" in order to meet "the nursing manpower needs of the future" (p. 256).

Benner, Sutphen, Leonard, and Day (2009) discuss the strengths and weaknesses in nursing education, and makes recommendations for programmatic educational changes and public policy reviews. Noting the separation that occurs between clinical and classroom teaching, Benner et al. (2009) recommends an integration of the two. Educators who are both faculty and practicing clinicians could more easily integrate didactic content with current clinical practice, closing that gap. In addition, masters and doctoral programs that are either clinically focused (DNP) or research focused (PhD) should include courses that prepare clinicians for the educator's role (Benner et al., 2009).

Collaborative arrangements can be accomplished in several ways. Part-time faculty appointments for selected specialty clinical experiences can be facilitated. For example, a pediatric nurse practitioner (PNP) interested in teaching pediatric nursing could be recruited to be a pediatric clinical instructor. Since this role most likely would not be a full-time position in an accelerated program of study, the advanced practice nurse (APN) could be hired as a part-time faculty member with reimbursement to the clinical agency for the time spent teaching. The APN may also elect to teach for additional compensation (i.e., teaching in the evenings or on weekends). Utilizing recognized clinical experts ensures clinically current education for nursing students. If the APN desires to teach more subjects than in one's identified specialty, one could be hired as a percent joint appointment and teach in health assessment and foundational skills labs. An arrangement as an official joint appointment with the school of nursing could be established where a percent appointment would be assigned for the school of nursing and the clinical practice site. This can increase the personal and professional satisfaction for the APN, allowing them the opportunity to impact on the future of nursing through educating nursing students while continuing on in their advanced practice role. These types of arrangements could assist in achieving an acceptable salary with the combined appointment. In *The Future of Nursing: Leading Change, Advancing Health* report from the Institute of Medicine (IOM, 2011), the salary disparities between nursing faculty and nurse practitioners are noted to be significant. The average salary for full-time nursing faculty is $64,949, as compared to nurse practitioners who average $85,000 (IOM, 2011). Faculty who hold nine-month appointments can spread out their teaching workload over 12 months, allowing for extra time to practice during the year. This income can be adjunctive to their faculty salary.

Recognizing the clinical expertise of staff nurses who are baccalaureate (BSN) prepared is also a way to recruit new faculty. Although it is essential to have faculty who are minimally master's (MSN) prepared as faculty teaching in an accelerated program, we need to identify a potential role for others in the academic program. Most clinical agencies, particularly those who have been recognized through American Nurses Credentialing Center (ANCC) Magnet Recognition Program®, have implemented clinical advancement systems for their nursing staff. For nurses who have been promoted within these advancement systems, clinical expertise and fostering education of new nurses is usually a part of the criteria for promotion. Working with the nursing administration of the practice setting, nurses can be selected for specific teaching roles within the academic program. The BS-prepared staff nurse could serve as assistant clinical teachers in a skills laboratory, working with MSN-prepared faculty for mentoring and supervision. This experience for the staff nurse may entice them to pursue advanced education, becoming our faculty of the future.

Maintaining contact with our most promising accelerated program graduates is another faculty recruitment possibility. Facilitating their involvement in the program as an assistant clinical teacher would serve two purposes. First, it would be inspirational for current students to see firsthand the success of the program's graduates and, second, this new role for the recent graduate may encourage them to pursue advanced education. Regardless of the purpose fulfilled, the assistant clinical teacher role could provide needed support for the laboratory faculty.

Faculty who are currently teaching in the accelerated programs can be the best recruiters for new faculty. If they are satisfied with their role, their salary, and the support of the school's administrators, they certainly will encourage others to apply for positions. It is imperative that attention is paid to current faculty to maximize their satisfaction, not only for them personally, but also for the role they can play in recruitment of others.

When recruiting an individual to assume a faculty position, it is essential that references on the individual are obtained and appropriate interviews are conducted. References need to address the person's interpersonal skills and professionalism as well as clinical competence; all are critical to fulfill the faculty role. Seasoned and novice faculty should both interview the applicant to ensure that an accurate understanding of faculty expectations is conveyed, while assessing the "goodness of fit" with the academic program.

Future Directions

Faculty recruitment should begin early, incorporating the roles and responsibilities of faculty in BS/BSN educational programs and focusing on the need for more faculty. Building excitement for the role that faculty play in the lives of those progressing through the profession can be accomplished in a variety of ways to facilitate early interest in a faculty career. Course offerings that focus on principles of adult learning and teaching of health professions should be standard elective offerings, either through an academic credit-bearing course or continuing education offerings. Valuing the role of faculty should clearly be articulated and demonstrated. Networking with clinical colleagues, focused recruitment initiatives, and strategic advertising will all enhance the recruitment of new faculty. Nursing faculty and advanced practice nurses need to advocate for financial compensation that is reflective of their credentials,

TABLE 9.1   Summary of Faculty Recruitment Challenges, Strategies, and Future Directions

CHALLENGES	STRATEGIES	FUTURE DIRECTIONS
Clinical and academic competence of faculty	Strategic marketing	Recruiting early in educational process
Faculty salaries	Collaborative affiliations with clinical agencies	Standardized course offerings
Requisite educational preparation of faculty	Recognition of clinically expert staff nurses Assistant clinical teachers	Advocate for elimination of salary disparities

experience, and expertise, regardless of the position that they hold (educator vs. practitioner). With the discrepancy in salary issues addressed in *The Future of Nursing* (IOM, 2011) report, this added attention will hopefully bring further discussion and recommendations to eliminate these disparities.

Table 9.1 summarizes the most significant faculty recruitment challenges, strategies, and future directions.

FACULTY RETENTION

Challenges

Successful recruitment strategies are for naught, if retention strategies are not consecutively implemented. Recognition of the challenges to retaining faculty must be considered. Salary disparities, working with demanding or difficult students, academic environment issues, and inflexible school administrators can all challenge faculty retention. Additionally, there are multiple opportunities for nurses with advanced degrees that will compete with the faculty role.

Implementing strategies to retain nursing faculty is critical for both novice and seasoned faculty, although the strategies may vary slightly. All faculty need to feel appreciated and valued and receive the support they need to teach within the program. Understanding what strategies will be most effective in retaining faculty is challenging, as individualized faculty needs are different and change over time. Strategies for faculty retention can be categorized into three areas: orientation programs, mentoring initiatives, and supportive approaches. Providing the financial resources for the implementation and ensuring time for participation in these activities can also be challenging.

Strategies

An orientation program for novice faculty or faculty new to the institution is vital to ensure adequate preparation prior to assuming the faculty role. Regardless of the format or the extent of the content presented, the implementation of an orientation program cannot be underestimated.

Pierangeli (2006) describes the development of a clinical teaching handbook and reference manual written for part-time faculty. The clinical teaching handbook could be utilized as a framework for an orientation program for all faculty. The handbook was developed with input from experienced faculty and included: information about the nursing department and university; successful teaching tips to use in the classroom and clinical setting; availability of school resources; choosing clinical assignments, conducting pre/post clinical conferences, and evaluating clinical performance; working with challenging students and the process of referral for additional supports; and, finally, various forms and samples of excellent student assignments are included (Pierangeli, 2006). Seasoned faculty should participate in the development of any orientation handbooks, including their feedback on content for inclusion. Encouraging their involvement demonstrates a respect and valuing of their expertise and experience, while ensuring that the essential components of the educational program are included.

Similar content as above was presented using a workshop format by Ellison and Williams (2009). The focus audience for this workshop was adjunct faculty but also included full-time faculty, with the goal of enhancing communication and increasing student success in their program. Both groups of faculty evaluated the workshops positively (Ellison & Williams, 2009).

An extensive process for educating new faculty was described by Bell-Scriber and Morton (2009) in their implementation of a grant supported by the Clinical Nursing Institute. The Institute was quite comprehensive, including a full-day introductory workshop, a three-credit graduate-level course, and ongoing mentoring. Evaluations from the participants were very positive, noting the benefits of ongoing mentoring, and access to clinical faculty who were experts in their field (Bell-Scriber & Morton, 2009). The comprehensiveness of this program might be cost-prohibited for schools to implement. Faculty would need to be compensated for attending the workshop and allotted time to attend the graduate course. In addition, mentoring of new faculty can be time intensive, possibly requiring additional compensation or adjustments/reduction in teaching workload. Aspects of the program could be initiated, however, with limited financial impact, specifically the full-day workshop and limiting the number of new faculty mentored by one seasoned faculty member.

Kalb (2008) noted that role components stated in the National League for Nursing's Core Competencies of Nurse Educators (National League for Nursing, 2005) can serve as the foundation for orientation of new faculty. The full range of roles and responsibilities for the nurse educator within an academic environment is important for new faculty to understand and appreciate (Kalb, 2008). Kalb (2008) also noted that faculty participation in self-evaluation can further assist in individualization of their orientation program. The more current faculty are involved in the development and implementation of an orientation program, the greater the likelihood of their retention and success in academia.

Mentoring of novice faculty by seasoned faculty can have reciprocal benefits and a formalized program can be instrumental in retaining faculty. Concern regarding significant faculty turnover at their institution led Alteen, Didham, and Stratton (2009) to develop a mentorship program to assist new faculty in their roles. The objectives of their program included development of faculty relationships, assistance with role transition, and utilization of seasoned faculty expertise and facilitation of a nurturing environment to promote development. Using an interactive workshop approach, activities were designed to encourage faculty to analyze and critique their current teaching pedagogies and approaches from various viewpoints. Their program was evaluated highly and demonstrated their commitment to the next generation of nurses (Alteen et al., 2009).

The Clinical Nursing Institute (Bell-Scriber & Morton, 2009) noted above also included a semester of mentored clinical instruction. The clinical coordinator of an individual course served as the identified mentor for any new faculty member and provided helpful hints for teaching while building a professional relationship. Frequent contacts and follow-up with the novice faculty assisted in providing assistance in a timely fashion (Bell-Scriber & Morton, 2009).

Blauvelt and Spath (2008) described a formal mentoring program as a strategy for faculty retention and designed in response to program expansion and the hiring of several new faculty. Their program was one year in length and focused on faculty development and retention. A mentoring handbook developed for the program contained information on mentoring, the faculty role, didactic and clinical course development, curriculum building and testing, and the role of advising. Since program implementation, 15 members of the faculty have participated. An eighty percent retention rate for new faculty was achieved with comments from the protégés, noting that "this program enabled them to not only survive but thrive in their first year of teaching" (Blauvelt & Spath, 2008, p. 32).

Regardless of the approach utilized, the importance of mentoring for novice and seasoned faculty is of utmost importance. Mentoring for seasoned faculty is often overlooked. As new pedagogies are introduced and more evidence-based teaching methodologies are explored, seasoned faculty may need to be mentored in new approaches. For example, with the introduction of information technology and simulated learning into schools of nursing, changes in pedagogy are needed. Seasoned faculty, who may have never learned to utilize these new approaches, can be mentored as they incorporate them into their clinical and didactic courses. Both seasoned and novice faculty teachers can learn together techniques on adopting new teaching methods facilitated by the latest technology. Learning together will enhance the satisfaction of all participants while facilitating professional development and fostering faculty retention.

In addition to formal orientation and mentoring programs, several strategies that support faculty (novice and seasoned) in their day-to-day process of teaching students can be implemented.

Ensuring that students have adequate resources to access (i.e., writing supports, math tutors, test-taking specialists, academic and clinical tutors), in addition to faculty teaching within the program, can ease the level of stress for faculty and students. Faculty feel supported knowing that there are additional services for student referral, minimizing the degree of burden they may feel for student success. When teaching large groups of accelerated students, it is difficult at times to focus on individual student needs; therefore, adding supplementary tutorial services is a welcomed addition.

Management of difficult or challenging students can also compound faculty stress and may cause them to "burn out." Faculty should feel encouraged to discuss these issues with course coordinators, program directors and/or senior nursing administrators. Role playing of common student scenarios or selected potential situations could begin during an orientation program as part of this process but then be individualized to meet the specific student situation.

Degree of faculty stress needs to be assessed and recognized, and often can be anticipated. Routine assessment of faculty satisfaction with specific attention to stressors should be conducted at least annually. Strategies for maximizing satisfaction can be jointly decided between the faculty member and school leadership and may include providing additional classroom supports (i.e., teaching assistants), more clinical mentorship, and/or joint problem solving "time."

Recognizing faculty for "going above and beyond," effectively managing a particular difficult situation, sharing expertise, or successful teaching/learning strategies with novice faculty, and so on, should be thoughtful and timely. This can be accomplished through electronic correspondence, a formal letter of recognition, or announcement at a faculty meeting or gathering. It should never go unnoticed! Bartels (2007) noted that new models of faculty awards should be advocated by school leadership and would "do wonders for morale and retention" (p. 157). In addition, as members of an academic community, we "need to learn that if we build a productive academic climate, they will come. If we support it, they will stay" (p. 158).

Recognition programs for faculty could include peer-nominated awards that acknowledge faculty for outstanding mentorship, creative teaching/learning strategies, professional collegiality, and clinical excellence. At the University of Rochester School of Nursing, faculty are recognized annually with faculty-nominated awards, including "Outstanding Faculty Colleague," "Outstanding Scholarly Practitioner," and a student-nominated, dean-selected award "Dean's Award for Excellence in Teaching." This latter award is presented to the faculty member at the annual graduation ceremony and includes a monetary gift. All methods of recognition are highlighted in a written annual report for the school, a school's newsletter, alumni publications, and spotlighted on the school's website. Each of these efforts demonstrates an appreciation for the time and energy our faculty commit to ensuring students' success.

Although the implementation of any of the above programs can be costly, the benefits of these far outweigh the costs and the return on investment. Faculty groups can be selected to work on the development of each activity (i.e., orientation/mentoring programs and supportive approaches), thus minimizing the associated workload. Involvement of faculty in each of these activities facilitates program ownership and promotes commitment to success. Schools should budget for expenses of each initiative, recognizing the cost of needing to hire replacement faculty would be much higher if programs for retention are not implemented.

Future Directions

Standardizing strategies to retain stellar faculty is the key to ensure that quality faculty are retained within the institution. There needs to be sincere thought and attention given to these initiatives, beginning with the assurance to incorporate any cost into the school's operating budget. The commitment must be transparent, involving as many faculty as possible in the process.

Yordy (2006) recommended several strategies to address the faculty shortage that can also assist in faculty retention, including:

- Establishment of a National Nursing Faculty Center to assist in supplying sources of data and expertise
- Creating a National Fellowship Program to facilitate faculty training and development and,
- Offering grants to support Centers of Excellence to assist in educating faculty (pp. 9, 10)

AACN (2005) suggested that an enhancement of the work environment for faculty and supportive faculty programs could assist in faculty retention. For example, creating an "Academies of Nurse Educators" whereby a core group of expert educators from the faculty would be identified with the goal of improving the faculty work environment and providing leadership and mentorship for the faculty may assist in faculty retention (p. 25).

As noted earlier, attention to faculty salaries, creating award recognition programs, and supportive administrative structures will also facilitate faculty retention; creativity in each of these areas is essential. The NLN Healthful Work Environment Toolkit (2006) could be utilized as an evaluative framework to assess areas of the work environment that may impact retention, for example, salaries/benefits, workload expectations, collegial environment, scholarship expectations and support, faculty development, and institutional support and recognition. Table 9.2 provides a summary of faculty retention challenges, strategies, and future directions.

TABLE 9.2 Summary of Faculty Retention Challenges, Strategies, and Future Directions

CHALLENGES	STRATEGIES	FUTURE DIRECTIONS
Varied effective strategies for novice and seasoned faculty	Orientation programs Mentoring initiatives	Standardized strategies Financing programs
Time for participation	Supportive approaches	Establishing new programs focused on retention strategies

FACULTY DEVELOPMENT

Challenges

Experienced and novice faculty both need continued professional development to meet the learning needs of our changing student population and academic programs. Understanding what the specific needs are and implementing appropriate learning activities can be challenging. Assessment of faculty development needs is critical to ensure that the most appropriate content is provided and that faculty needs are addressed.

Strategies

Recognizing common faculty educational needs can assist in building an effective faculty development program. Creating a formal process is essential, particularly for faculty members who have not received formal educational preparation in teaching (Bartels, 2007).

There are numerous educational topics and methods that will aid in developing faculty. *Understanding the accelerated nursing student.* It is essential to recognize the differences between generic undergraduate students and the accelerated nursing student and strategies to promote their success. Mangold (2007) noted the challenges for faculty who are "baby-boomers" teaching students with significant generational differences—"millennial students" (p. 21). Educational activities for faculty should include strategies for teaching students who are more technologically savvy, proficient at multitasking, favor interactional teaching/ learning strategies and may value "doing" over "knowing" (Mangold, 2007). The accelerated student has different learning needs than the traditional baccalaureate student as their previous education and experience creates a new lens for learning. For example, a student with a prior degree in chemistry or biochemistry will learn laboratory test interpretation and its application to the clinical setting with more in-depth focus. In addition, the accelerated student may have an established learning pattern that may not be congruent with clinical nursing education. Hands-on learning, psychomotor skill development, simulated learning experiences, case-based/problem-based learning are common teaching/learning strategies for students in a nursing program in which other students may lack familiarity. This can be anxiety producing for the new nursing student learner.

Nontraditional Teaching Strategies

Faculty-directed learning that "tells" students what they need to learn without involving the student in the learning process is rarely an acceptable teaching strategy, especially for the accelerated nursing student. Collaboration with clinical agencies can provide resources to facilitate this educational process. Educators experienced in staff development are often quite skilled in nontraditional teaching strategies and can assist in faculty development (Mathews, 2003). Problem-based learning techniques, use of simulation, student-led seminars, and case-based approaches are common strategies for teaching that may be new to novice and new faculty, and in some cases to even experienced faculty. Educational offerings provided by experts in a variety of these teaching/learning techniques are essential to incorporate in faculty development workshops. Observations of current faculty with expertise in various teaching methodologies and formal mentoring for skill acquisition would help others to add to their own repertoire of educational strategies. Teaching sessions utilizing different techniques could be recorded and viewed by others for learning purposes and to critique strengths and weaknesses of each approach.

Developing a Philosophy of Teaching

Whether or not we articulate our philosophy to one another or are conscious of our own philosophy, most faculty do have a guiding philosophical premise to teaching. Sweitzer (2003) comments on the process of promoting reflectivity as a way to nurture faculty development. A "reflective professor" has a philosophy that includes beliefs about teaching and learning, goals, students, and themselves. A development activity for faculty could include the composition of individualized teaching philosophies, helping faculty to reflect upon the pros and cons of each. Similar to the importance of clinicians learning and implementing a philosophy of caring and clinical practice, a philosophy of teaching informs and guides the practice of education. It is imperative that educators have a conceptual foundation from which to teach that will guide their teaching/learning strategies, interactions with students and evaluation processes. Students in an accelerated program, who hold undergraduate and/or graduate degrees in another field, already have experienced the higher-education system and have been exposed to a variety of educators. For example, some of these students may have experienced faculty who "impart" knowledge, while others may have encountered those that are "facilitators" of knowledge. Understanding the difference in educational philosophies and how the differences impact on the experience of learning is critical for the novice as well as a seasoned faculty member.

Characteristics of Effective Teachers

Although some faculty may be quite established in their approaches to teaching or ways of interacting with students, it is always refreshing (and enlightening at times) to share current research on perceptions of effective teachers. Focused attention should be given to interpersonal characteristics of effective vs. ineffective teachers (Berg & Lindseth, 2004; Mangold, 2007; Tang, Chou, & Chiang, 2005; Wolf, Bender, Beitz, Wieland, & Vito, 2004) to further emphasize the importance of developing a supportive learning environment. Berg and Lindseth (2004) noted several characteristics of the effective teacher that could enhance the environment for learning. Effective teachers are approachable, easy to communicate with, respectful, concerned, patient, and fair (Berg & Lindseth, 2004). Demonstrating these characteristics (and the opposites as well) through role plays or simulated faculty–student scenarios could assist in illustrating the positive and negative impact of each on the educational milieu.

Conducting Clinical Evaluations

Often, the subjective premise of clinical evaluations makes the process of evaluating students challenging. Providing an evaluation using sensitive, yet clear communication skills, is an art that is cultivated over time. Mahara and Jones (2005) noted that "becoming skillful at clinical evaluations requires experience, reflection, and collaboration with peers" (p. 129) and utilized a participative inquiry approach for teaching this process. Presenting positive feedback with suggestions for improvement and/or issues of concern needs to be balanced and the techniques for doing so need to be practiced. Students who "hear" only the negatives may not learn from the evaluation process, thereby negating its purpose. Summarizing a student's strengths and incorporating strategies for future success with skills in need of improvement will ensure a more effective and constructive evaluation. This core education provided to faculty will demystify the evaluation process and allow them the opportunity to "rehearse" a meaningful evaluation. It is also appropriate to have a seasoned faculty member accompany a novice faculty member during a "live" student evaluation meeting to provide support during the actual process. Afterwards, both faculty could critique the process and discuss methods for improvement as needed.

Curriculum Building and Test Construction

Developing, implementing, and evaluating curriculum is a critical process that requires significant understanding of accreditation standards, *The Essentials of Baccalaureate Education for Professional Nursing Practice* (AACN, 2008), and state regulatory requirements and NCLEX test plans. Specific education about and practice with curriculum design and implementation and test construction is requisite knowledge to ensure a high-quality, rigorous educational program. Content on how to write measurable course and clinical objectives, level objectives for advancing knowledge, perform content mapping and analyze results to inform curricular modifications, assess knowledge and skill acquisition, and evaluate competence need to be considered. While the basics of this content can be taught initially, the actual process of "doing" is the best method of instruction for this content. As new courses are developed or current courses revised, novice faculty can be exposed to this process and mentored.

Evaluating Student-Learning Outcomes

Accrediting agencies and institutes of higher education have become increasingly focused on ensuring that student learning outcomes are identified, assessed, and utilized as measurements of student success. Educating faculty on these processes is essential for the development of a solid curriculum and for effective evaluation of student learning outcomes. Paramount to this process is the involvement of faculty in determining what program and student outcomes are of most importance to their particular program. It is essential for faculty to discuss the "purposes" for their course/program of study and what they want the learners to be able to "do" at the completion of the course/program. Determining student learning outcomes cannot be an afterthought but should be discussed from the beginning. As outcomes are determined and agreed upon, the next focus needs to be on the "how to" of measuring if the outcome has been achieved. A variety of outcome measures, both qualitative and quantitative, should be employed with careful attention as to the process of evidence gathering and analysis. Critical to the process of student learning outcome assessment and evaluation is "closing the loop." As outcomes are measured and analyzed, any outcome not meeting a threshold for success will need to be reviewed to determine the factors impacting on success and steps taken to ensure improvement. Recommendations for improvement should include both faculty and students, as both groups are key to program quality and success.

TABLE 9.3 Summary of Faculty Development Challenges, Strategies, and Future Directions

CHALLENGES	STRATEGIES	FUTURE DIRECTIONS
Varied needs of novice and seasoned faculty	Formal process for assessment	Standardized assessment
Assessment of faculty development needs	Topics for consideration Methods of providing development opportunities	Identification of lead faculty

Future Directions

Assessing faculty developmental needs must be a continual process, particularly as new faculty members are recruited and seasoned faculty members retire. This can be accomplished through formal surveys conducted at least annually and individually during annual performance evaluations. A variety of methods can be employed to provide the professional development assessed as needed by the faculty. Development retreats with featured educational experts, series of educational workshops, online offerings or "teaching hours" could be offered. Identifying an individual to lead these efforts within each institution or creating an Office for Faculty Development facilitates concentrated attention to its importance.

As more accelerated nursing programs are developed and implemented, the recruitment, retention and development of faculty for these programs is the key to their continued success. Purposeful attention to each is issue is vital to ensuring that a quality educational program is not only maintained but also continues to advance our profession. Table 9.3 summarizes faculty development challenges, strategies, and future directions.

CONCLUSION

Focused attention to faculty recruitment, retention, and development is critical to attaining and maintaining a highly qualified faculty. The faculty shortage is real, particularly with our aging faculty workforce, increasing workload demand and less than robust salary packages. Encouraging nurses to enter faculty roles earlier, combining faculty appointments with clinical practice appointments, creating flexible workload assignments, and advocating for increased salary support are all effective strategies to increase faculty recruitment. Retaining faculty in their current positions requires an understanding of the issues of importance for each faculty member. Providing a structured orientation program, institution of mentoring initiatives, supporting faculty with resources for success, and rewarding faculty accomplishments are critical for faculty retention. Faculty development programs for both novice and seasoned faculty will ensure ongoing assessment of faculty needs and support the critical development of both groups. Schools of nursing need to be proactive in their approaches for recruitment, retention, and development of faculty to ensure the future of our profession.

REFERENCES

AACN. (2005). *Faculty shortages in baccalaureate and graduate nursing programs: Scope of the problem and strategies for expanding the supply.* Washington, DC: Author.

AACN. (2008). *The essentials of baccalaureate education for professional nursing practice.* Washington, DC: Author.

Alteen, A. M., Didham, P., & Stratton, C. (2009). Reflecting, refueling, and reframing: A 10-year retrospective model for faculty development and its implications for nursing scholarship. *The Journal of Continuing Education in Nursing, 40*(6), 267–272.

Bartels, J. E. (2007). Preparing nursing faculty for baccalaureate-level and graduate-level nursing programs: Role preparation for the academy. *Journal of Nursing Education, 46*(4), 154–158.

Bell-Scriber, M. J., & Morton, A. M. (2009). Clinical instruction: Train the trainer. *Nurse Educator, 34*(2), 84–87.

Benner, P., Sutphen, M., Leonard, V., & Day, L. (2009) *Educating nurses: A call for radical transformation.* San Francisco: Jossey-Bass.

Berg, C. L., & Lindseth, G. (2004). Students' perspectives of effective and ineffective nursing instructors. *Journal of Nursing Education, 43*(12), 565–568.

Blauvelt, M. J., & Spath, M. L. (2008). Passing the torch: A faculty mentoring program at one school of nursing. *Nursing Education Perspectives, 29*(4), 29–33.

Ellison, D., & Williams, M. (2009). Implementing an orientation/mentorship program for adjunct faculty. *The Tennessee Nurse*, p.5.

IOM (Institute of Medicine). (2011). *The future of nursing: Leading change, advancing health.* Washington, DC: The National Academies Press.

Kalb, K. A. (2008). Core competencies of nurse educators: Inspiring excellence in nurse educator practice. *Nurse Education Perspectives, 29*(4), 217–219.

Kaufman, K. (2007). Introducing the NLN/Carnegie National Survey of Nurse Educators: Compensation, workload, and teaching practice. *Nursing Education Perspectives, 28*(3), 164–168.

Kaufman, K. A. (2009). *Executive summary: Findings from the 2009 Faculty Census.* Retrieved from; http://www.nln.org/research/slides/fc_exec_summary0809.pdf

Mahara, M. S., & Jones, J. A. (2005). Participatory inquiry with a colleague: An innovative faculty development process. *Journal of Nursing Education, 44*(3), 124–130.

Mangold, K. (2007). Educating a new generation: Teaching baby boomer faculty about millennial students. *Nurse Educator, 32*(1), 21–23.

Mathews, M. B. (2003). Resourcing nursing education through collaboration. *The Journal of Continuing Education in Nursing, 34*(6), 251–257.

National League for Nursing. (2005). *Core competencies of nurse educators with task statements.* Retrieved from http://www.nln.org/facultydevelopment/pdf/corecompetencies.pdf

National League for Nursing. (2006). *National League for Nursing: Healthful work environment tool kit*©. New York: Author.

Pierangeli, L. (2006). Developing a clinical teaching handbook and reference manual for part-time clinical faculty. *Nurse Educator, 31*(4), 183–185.

Sweitzer, H. F. (2003). Getting off to a good start: Faculty development in professional programs. *The Journal of Continuing Education in Nursing, 34,* 263–272.

Tang, F., Chou, S., & Chiang, H. (2005). Students' perceptions of effective and ineffective clinical instructors. *Journal of Nursing Education, 44*(4), 187–192.

Wolf, Z. R., Bender, P. J., Beitz, J. M., Wieland, D. M., & Vito, K. O. (2004). Strengths and weaknesses of faculty teaching performance reported by undergraduate and graduate nursing students: A descriptive study. *Journal of Professional Nursing, 20*(2), 118–128.

Yordy, K. D. (2006). *The Nursing faculty shortage: A crisis for health care.* Washington, DC: Robert Wood Johnson Foundation.

Chapter 10

Educational Resources for Accelerated Nursing Programs: Challenges, Strategies, and Future Directions

Linda M. Caldwell and Susan A. LaRocco

P rior to creating an accelerated nursing program, many decisions must be made about the resources necessary to establish a successful program. Better resources for faculty, staff, and budget have been linked to improved student retention and program quality (Ari, 2009) and therefore it is extremely important to consider which resources are essential, which would be useful, and which can be discarded or denied. At this time of fiscal restraint necessitated by the global economic downturn, it may be difficult to establish a new nursing program unless the program generates more revenue than the expenses it will incur. It is also very likely that resource requests from faculty will outnumber available finances in today's academic climate. Consideration must also be given to the accreditation requirements and recommendations for resources of the National League for Nursing Accrediting Commission (NLNAC) or the Commission on Collegiate Nursing Education (CCNE); expansion of programs and/or students may require expansion of resources for continuing accreditation. In addition, state boards of nursing and state departments of education may have their own regulations and mandates for required or recommended resources for a new program.

Critical questions need to be answered as a school plans for resource acquisition for any new educational offering. While each nursing school has unique issues and challenges, some common and basic decisions must be made in the early stages of program development. When the Division of Nursing at Curry College designed an accelerated nursing program we considered the following questions:

- Will the accelerated program be a second-degree baccalaureate program or a direct-entry master's program?
- Will it be a day program or convene on an evening and/or weekend schedule?
- Will some of the courses be taught online or as hybrid courses?
- What is the maximum number of students that can be accommodated? What are the constraining factors for this number?
- Will more faculty members be needed, or are current faculty sufficient and qualified?
- Are there sufficient clinical placements available? When are they available—during the Monday to Friday academic schedule or only on an alternate schedule such as weekends or evenings?
- Should the program continue through the summer or should it only be offered during the traditional academic year?
- What will be the impact on faculty scheduling and workload if the program runs during the summer?
- Can a summer session be part of a faculty member's contractual work load?

While these questions will generate an initial discussion, there will be many opportunities to revisit the answers as the program planning phase continues and as the resources, or lack thereof, become apparent.

Assumptions in this chapter are that an accelerated baccalaureate program will be an addition to an existing traditional prelicensure nursing program. As such, many of the basic resources, such as nursing labs and library holdings, will already exist. The focus of this chapter will be on the necessary expansion of resources to accommodate the additional students in the accelerated program whose needs are often different from the typical undergraduate. Areas to be discussed include clinical affiliations, faculty numbers and preparation, teaching and learning environment resources, technology, and funding for the program.

CLINICAL AFFILIATIONS

Clinical affiliations are an important component of any nursing program. In accelerated nursing education, with the shortened time span, appropriate clinical placements become more significant than they are in a lengthier traditional program. Providing the students with a variety of experiences is crucial to their future success as nurses. In many areas of the country, clinical placements are becoming more difficult to find. Expanding enrollments have increased the competition among schools of nursing for high-quality clinical sites. With the introduction of an accelerated program, faculty may find that they are also competing with their own traditional baccalaureate program for the same clinical sites. This is especially true in the specialty areas such as pediatrics, maternity, and mental health nursing.

Because of increased patient acuity, decreased length of stay, and concerns about quality and safety, some hospitals are decreasing the student-to-faculty ratio, not only in specialty areas but also in general medical surgical units. A recent decision by Massachusetts General Hospital in Boston to decrease clinical group size from eight to six is typical of this trend. This results in a need for not only more clinical sites, but also more clinical faculty. In addition to the strain on resources, the cost of education will of necessity increase. Availability of clinical placements may force the decision to run the program during evening and weekend hours.

Decisions about the scheduling of clinical hours also need to be made. Should there be an immersion experience at the end of the program? How long should the clinical day be? With many hospitals using 12-hour shift scheduling, is that an appropriate model for students as well?

In the clinical setting it is also important to select sites with the right atmosphere. Accelerated second-degree students are typically older than traditional students and have many skills and life experience. However, they are novices in the patient care setting. Encouraging the staff in the clinical setting to value the experience of the adult learner while still assisting them to become proficient nurses may pose a challenge (Caldwell, Tenofsky, & Nugent, 2010). In many cases the student will be working with a nurse who is years younger than the student. This may cause conflict and inhibit effective working relationships (Keepnews, Brewer, Kovner, & Shin, 2010).

In terms of additional resources for the program, there may need to be time allocated for orientation to adult learning theory for the clinical faculty and perhaps for the staff at the clinical site. Faculty who are comfortable teaching traditional students may have difficulty transitioning to meeting the needs of adult learners. Characteristics of adult learners include:

- A need to know why they need to learn something
- A need to learn in a more experiential style
- A preference for a problem-solving approach to learning

■ Most engaged when they perceive the topic to have immediate value (Knowles et al., 2005)

FACULTY RESOURCES

Determining the faculty resources needed for an accelerated program is much more than calculating workload requirements and student–faculty ratios. Several basic decisions need to be made as the program is developed. One question that needs to be answered is whether the faculty assigned to the accelerated program will be dedicated to that program or if faculty who currently teach in the traditional program will be assigned to both programs. The contractual environment must also be considered. If the program will run during the summer, will faculty be allowed to use summer teaching as part of their regular academic workload? Will full-time faculty want to be available during the summer or will much of the summer teaching be done by adjunct faculty? Will additional full-time faculty be needed to accommodate the expanded enrollment? When considering faculty costs, benefits must also be considered and will typically add another 25–30% to the compensation cost for new full-time faculty. Undoubtedly, additional part-time faculty will be needed.

In addition to faculty time for teaching, creation of a new program will likely result in allocating faculty time to administer the program. There has to be some monetary provision allowed for administration and leadership of the program. If the school has a faculty union, early involvement of the union leadership regarding titles and time allocation while planning the program can prevent difficulties later in the approval process. The amount of time needed for program coordination and leadership will depend on what aspects of the program are the responsibilities of the nursing unit. If the program is housed in a continuing education department, questions about responsibility for various aspects of the program must be decided during the development stage. Areas that need to be discussed include who staffs information sessions, responds to inquiries, processes applications, and screens for health and other clinical clearances. If the nursing unit is expected to manage any of these responsibilities, time allocation for faculty and support staff must be factored into the program budget. The addition of a new program can easily strain the resources of a nursing unit if these details are not discussed and planned for prior to the recruitment of the first class. If these tasks are managed by another department, nursing faculty time must be allocated for coordinating with that department and updating them on the frequent changes needed for students to be admitted to clinical settings. The requirements for clinical contracts, health clearances, background checks, and constraints on the number of students in a clinical agency are foreign to other academic departments, and the college administration may also find them hard to understand. The leadership in the nursing department needs to be able to fluently articulate to the college administration why these requirements are needed in order to obtain the fiscal resources to cover the associated costs.

Cangelosi and Moss (2010) studied faculty who were teaching accelerated students. Using hermeneutic phenomenology, they sought to "understand the meaning of the everyday experiences of faculty teaching accelerated second degree baccalaureate students" (p. 138). The two themes that emerged from their interviews with 14 nursing faculty were labeled "at the top of my game" and "teaching to think like a nurse." Faculty, particularly novice teachers, indicated that the accelerated students could be intimidating because they challenge teachers by pointing out obscure details. Students were also described as inquisitive, demanding, and perfectionists. Some faculty, especially those who have only taught traditional college-age students, may find the transition to second-degree students difficult and somewhat frustrating. Workshops, team teaching, and peer review of classes may be helpful, particularly for the novice teacher. Education on adult learning theory may be helpful and may be provided economically by asking the education faculty in the college for assistance with workshops. The American Association of Colleges of Nursing (AACN) also offers helpful webinars for faculty development on a variety of topics throughout the academic year.

TEACHING AND LEARNING ENVIRONMENT RESOURCES

The teaching and learning environment for the accelerated student presents challenges and opportunities in a variety of ways. In the classroom, faculty may be tempted to lecture and "get through" a vast amount of material. However, the adult learner may be on his laptop or smart phone searching out information as the lecture continues and may challenge the professor with information he has found. Opportunities for the classroom to have ready access to reliable sources of Internet-based medical, nursing, and health information should be available and the teaching faculty members need to know how to use the technology with ease. Multiple LCDs and screens are ideal tools for this type of classroom environment. Personal response systems, in which the student immediately answers questions using an electronic device, are another way to keep the adult learner engaged with the topic under discussion (Revell and McCurry, 2010).

Both systems require an initial investment in terms of capital outlay and faculty orientation to use the devices effectively.

Class scheduling is another area to consider. Adult learners, with multiple other responsibilities, appreciate having trips to campus for classroom instruction and clinical experiences minimized. Scheduling classes over one or two days decreases the commuting time, but increases the information load for the day. That trade-off must be considered. Alternating types of courses, for example, scheduling an intense adult acute care course followed by a research or health policy course might mitigate the overload. The classroom environment itself needs to be considered. Having a dedicated classroom where all classes are held may lead to a sense of belonging and familiarity, but having a change of environment during the day might be needed to prevent environmental fatigue. An example of a strategy to prevent this fatigue is to intersperse lab time and simulated experiences with traditional class lectures. This will help to keep students engaged in learning through a long day by frequent refocusing of physical and mental activity.

Students in an accelerated program may be competing with other nursing programs in the school for use of laboratory space. If labs are a required component of the accelerated curriculum, scheduling those lab classes may decrease the amount of "non-scheduled lab time" or available open-access lab time for students in all programs to practice skills or become familiar with equipment. Scheduling of lab time may be particularly problematic in programs that have seen recent expansion in enrollment without a corresponding increase in lab space. Coordination when scheduling labs among programs is necessary so that two lab classes are not scheduled at the same time. Which program has priority for lab time and space may become a significant issue among faculty.

Staffing the lab with faculty who have both an interest in the lab and who can be available when the accelerated students are available can be a particular challenge. Lab staffing may be accommodated with faculty hours or by lab staff paid at an hourly rate. A blended position, with the lab faculty serving as faculty some of the time and in staff positions paid at an hourly rate at other times is another option. The lab hours for instruction and the lab hours where the lab is open to students need to be calculated and the best method of staffing the lab selected. Some consistency of staff/faculty in the lab is desirable, particularly when simulators are used. Skill and competency testing also require lab faculty and subsequently will increase expenditures.

Dennison (2010) discussed peer mentoring as a valuable and often overlooked resource. While she describes the clear benefits for both mentors and mentees in a traditional program, the same benefits would likely accrue in a mentoring relationship between traditional and accelerated students. Mentees described feeling less intimidated with a mentor while learning new skills than when they were with a faculty member. Peer mentors can provide individualized attention and a more relaxed environment than would be possible with limited faculty time.

TECHNOLOGY

Globalization of health care, availability of instant information to patients, rapid advances in technology, multiple and frequent changes in the health care system, and the changing demographics of patients currently converge to create a constant demand for ever more expensive and sophisticated technology. As the nursing profession becomes more focused on quality, safety, team work, and evidence, simulation in the lab becomes a priority to enhance learning while allowing students to make errors in a safe environment where no harm will befall a patient. High-fidelity simulators are becoming more of an expectation for prospective students in every type of nursing program. Although the high-fidelity simulators are quite expensive, grants may be obtained to help with the purchase. Low-fidelity simulators are less expensive and can also be used to provide simulated clinical experiences. When planning for simulation, time for faculty to learn to use the equipment should be factored into the budget. The learning curve for the high-fidelity simulators is steep, but a simulator that is not used may as well have not been purchased. A "faculty champion" may need to be selected to keep abreast of technology advances and to update other faculty members on what is available and how to effectively utilize the new technology. Clinical adjuncts will need orientation to the college system for grade submission and to access the associated theory course.

While some accelerated students may have skills in technology that surpass faculty, others are technologically naive. Certainly, both groups have different needs but both may need an orientation to the course delivery system used in the program, such as Blackboard or e-courseware. Orientation for class and clinical faculty to use course technology must be considered and planned for as well.

Another aspect of technology involves library resources. Students who are not on campus on a daily basis expect to have off-site access to library databases, including full-text journal articles and electronic books. As this is common in college libraries, it should not require any additional resources for a new nursing program. However, current financial challenges may reduce budget allocations to the library, despite the fact that the demand is for more library holdings as health care knowledge expands and evolves.

PROGRAM FUNDING

In tuition-driven colleges and universities, the revenue generated from the programming should cover the associated expenses. If the program is initiated by grant funding, sustainability of both the grant, and ultimately of the program, needs to be carefully weighed.

Program expenses will include time for initial planning and then marketing the program. The most significant cost center will be for additional full- and part-time faculty salaries and benefits and the expenses associated with nonfaculty personnel, such as administrative assistant time and personnel to handle the processing of applications. If applicants are to be interviewed prior to admission, time and money need to be budgeted for the interviewers. Costs associated with any consultants that might be needed should be included as well. Additional other program expenditures are shown in Exhibit 10.1.

It is important to consider that financial aid for second baccalaureate program students may not be available if students have "tapped out" their limit on financial aid for their prior undergraduate program. Loans may be necessary for students to be able to finance the program. The federal nursing scholarship program may be available to students who are willing to commit to future service in an underserved area. Information may be obtained from the Health Resources and Services Administration web site (www.hrsa.gov).

SUMMARY

Although resources are an important aspect of program planning, a vision for the program in terms of size and structure must be decided prior to considering resources for a new program. It is extremely important to consider which resources are essential and which are not. Remember that desired resources will likely exceed available finances.

Clinical sites must be carefully selected to provide an opportunity for accelerated students to learn in an environment that is challenging yet nurturing. Lab and classroom space should be designated with consideration of the existing programs so that the allocations are complementary rather than competitive. Technology can be a huge financial drain. Selection of equipment, simulators, and media should be made carefully, with an eye

---

EXHIBIT 10.1   ADDITIONAL PROGRAM EXPENDITURES

Accreditation costs

State-approval expenses

College fairs for recruitment

Supplies and administrative staff

Associated clinical expenses (contracts, legal fees, etc.)

Faculty mileage and parking if paid by the school

Advising events

Office furniture and supplies for additional staff and/or faculty

Lab expenses such as extra lab supplies and equipment

Media expenses

Computerized tests if used in the program

Outcome surveys—such as Educational Benchmarking Inc.

Graduation events

TABLE 10.1   Educational Resources Challenges, Strategies, and Future Directions in Accelerated Nursing Programs

CHALLENGES	STRATEGIES	RESOURCES
Assuring that there are adequate clinical sites and qualified faculty are the most significant challenges for a new accelerated program Preparing clinical and academic faculty to teach adult learners who are highly motivated and often demanding can also be challenging Balancing the needs of existing programs with the new program can be difficult	Consider scheduling clinical experiences during the summer or on weekends or evenings to allow for a larger choice of clinical sites Provide adequate orientation regarding the differences of adult learners for all full- and part-time faculty who will be teaching in the program As much as possible, schedule faculty who want to work with the second-degree students Discuss need for both programs with faculty and staff who will teach in the various programs	Accelerated programs will continue to grow in size and number as the anticipated shortage of nurses continues Students who enter these programs will continue to be more focused and challenging to faculty, but will add to the nursing work force and make significant contributions, and may become the nursing faculty of the future Competition for resources such as faculty, lab time, and classroom space for each program within a nursing school and between nursing schools will exacerbate

for utility over time, and potential impact on the curriculum. Frequent advances in technology and frequent changes in the health care system create a constant demand for ever more expensive and sophisticated technology. The need for faculty to keep pace with technological advances is imperative, as are the associated expenses. As personnel costs of faculty and administrative staff will likely be the largest expense of a new program, all factors associated with hiring of new personnel need to be considered. A summary of challenges, strategies, and future directions in educational resources for accelerated nursing programs is shown in Table 10.1.

REFERENCES

Ari, A. (2009). Connecting students to institutions: The relationship between program resources and student retention in respiratory care education programs. *Respiratory Care, 54*(9), 1187–1192.

Caldwell, L. M., Tenofsky, L. M., & Nugent, E. (2010). Academic and clinical immersion in an ACCELERATED nursing program to foster learning in the adult student. *Nursing Education Perspectives, 31*(5), 294–297.

Cangelosi, P. R., & Moss, M. M. (2010). Voices of faculty of second-degree baccalaureate nursing students. *Journal of Nursing Education, 4*(3), 137–142.

Dennison, S. (2010). Peer mentoring: Untapped potential. *Journal of Nursing Education, 49*(6), 340–342.

Keepnews, D. M., Brewer, C. S., Kovner, C. T., & Shin, J. H. (2010). Generational differences among newly licensed registered nurses. *Nursing Outlook, 58*(3), 155–163.

Knowles, M. S., Holton, III, E. F., & Swanson, R. A. (2005). *The Adult Learner* (6th ed.) Burlington, MA: Elsevier.

Revell, S. M., & McCurry, M. K. (2010). Engaging millennial learners: Effectiveness of personal response system technology with nursing students in small and large classrooms. *Journal of Nursing Education, 49*(5), 272–275.

Accelerated Nursing Education: Interprofessional Approach

Chapter

11

Accelerated Education in Radiologic Sciences: A Broader Perspective

Lisa Fanning, Frances K. Keech, and Susan B. Belinsky

INTRODUCTION

*I*n 2002, a program conversion was made to change the traditional 4-year bachelors in radiologic science degree (radiation therapy, nuclear medicine technology, and radiography) to a 3-year accelerated format to potentially increase the enrollment within a competitive environment. The accelerated programs offered at the college are defined as a shortened program of study, typically 3 years, awarding a bachelor of science in radiologic sciences with a major in nuclear medicine technology, radiography, or radiation therapy. This is a shortened time period in comparison with a traditional 4-year degree program. The authors' experience described in this chapter is derived from their analysis of admissions and student assessment data, curriculum changes, and programmatic outcomes.

AN OVERVIEW

Accelerated programs have become more popular within colleges over time in the United States. There are several factors that account for the increase in accelerated programs. According to *The New York Times* (Honan, 1993), the California higher-education state system is using an accelerated approach to undergraduate degrees, mainly as a cost-saving strategy to the students and a means of dealing with increasing enrollment and a decline in funding from the state system. Private colleges see this as a means to increase retention instead of students finishing their education at a less costly public institution. Preparatory schools see this as an opportunity for growth as they prepare students for these accelerated programs.

There is no compilation of statistics available that looks at accelerated programs across the field of allied health such as radiological sciences. These programs do exist, but they are very few in number specifically in the field of radiologic sciences. Bates College located in Brunswick, Maine, was the first higher-educational institution in the United States to offer a liberal arts degree in an accelerated format in 1965 (Shellenbarger, 2010).

Utilizing the Joint Review Committee in Education of Radiologic Technology (JRCERT) and Joint Review Committee of Nuclear Medicine Technology (JRCNMT) databases, it was concluded that eight accelerated radiologic science programs exist in the United States, including the three programs currently available at the Massachusetts College of Pharmacy and Health Sciences (MCPHS). Although five other programs claim to be accelerated, they do not follow the format for a true accelerated education. The true accelerated program is one in which students enter into the college without requiring any prerequisite courses. All required courses are built into the program of study. To date, the only existing programs that follow the accelerated program model in Radiologic Sciences are those at MCPHS. According to the JRCERT and JRCNMT databases, there are 109 accredited nuclear medicine technology programs, 636 accredited radiography programs, and 82 accredited radiation therapy programs.

In comparison with nursing programs, the American Association of Colleges of Nursing (AACN, 2010) reports there were 230 Bachelor Science of Nursing (BSN) accelerated programs out of the 1500 total BSN programs across the country. The total number has increased from 31 in 1990. Table 11.1 presents data for accelerated radiological sciences programs.

DIFFERENCES BETWEEN UNITED STATES AND INTERNATIONAL ACCELERATED PROGRAMS

Accelerated education is not a new concept. Many European countries and Australia have used this model. High schools in these countries emphasize career development by offering students in their final 2 years

TABLE 11.1   Accelerated Radiological Sciences Program Statistics

TYPE OF PROGRAM	PERCENTAGE OF ACCELERATED PROGRAMS	TOTAL NUMBER OF PROGRAMS
NURSING	15.33	1500
Radiologic sciences:		
Nuclear medicine technology	0.91	109
Radiography	0.16	636
Radiation therapy	1.21	82
Totals	0.36	827

of school exposure to their field of interest. During this time, students are allowed to take courses relative to their potential careers. These 2 years introduce coursework that is equivalent to first-year college studies in the United States. They also have opportunities to observe professionals in their prospective fields. As a result of this career development experience, students enter universities better prepared for the profession they would like to pursue.

Not only have these countries been successful with the 3-year model, but also the European Union (EU) has elected to continue in this format and maintain competitiveness with the United States. In addition, they have adopted a consistent design across all its member countries. This initiative, named the "Bologna Process," was designed to construct uniformity across the borders of 46 countries in the European Union; one educational objective is to create a seamless degree granting process in higher education (Morgan, 2010). This process essentially integrates the EU higher-educational system by:

- Creating frameworks for national qualifications and learning outcomes for all higher-education levels and "easily readable, comparable degrees."
- Aligning Standards and Guidelines for Quality Assurance in European Higher Education Area.
- Recognizing foreign degrees and other higher-education qualifications in accordance with the Council of Europe/UNESCO Recognition Convention (European Commission Education and Training, 2011).

In contrast to the United States, the majority of European students do not have these career development internships unless they attend either a vocational technical or career-centered high school (magnet) that trains students for specific careers such as medical, dental lab assistant, or nursing assistant (Health Career Center, 2011). The transition from a high school to a college may be more difficult since the high-school curriculum may not focus on a concentration of interest as compared to the international experience. Typically accelerated college programs with their more demanding academics and more concentrated curricula are geared toward enrolling motivated students. From the authors' combined 37 years of experience in higher education, they have observed that the motivated students have taken advanced placement or honor courses in high school. Some students who have taken advanced placement courses are allowed to transfer these credits into the higher-education institution, giving them some relief from the rigors of the condensed curriculum in an accelerated program (Honan, 1993). Table 11.2 compares U.S., European, and Australian Accelerated Programs.

MCPHS Accelerated Curriculum. To accommodate the 3-year format student core and professional classes are compressed into eight semesters. The minimal numbers of credits are typically 16–18 credits per spring and fall semesters, and 9–12 credits in the summer. The school's fall and spring semesters are 15 weeks in length. The summer semesters vary between 5 and 12 weeks. An example of the first year curriculum for accelerated radiologic science majors is shown in Table 11.3.

Year one, students begin taking general prerequisite courses in the fall semester. The professional course work commences in the summer of that first year. They then complete six continuous semesters of academics and clinical internships until the end of spring in the 3rd year. The decision to make the change from the previous 4-year format was based on a recruitment strategy to increase radiologic science enrollment, and to counter multiple competing associate degree programs within a small geographic area. These associate degree granting colleges provide a 2-year format. However, in most cases, students are required to fulfill a number of

TABLE 11.2 The United States, Europe, and Australian Accelerated Program Length/Transition Methods Comparisons

	UNITED STATES	EUROPE AND AUSTRALIA
Program length	■ Majority of higher institution programs: 4 years	■ Majority of higher institution programs: 3 years
Transitioning methods	■ Transition is better suited for motivated high school students or students who attended career-oriented high schools	■ Students in their final 2 years of high school concentrate on a field of interest
		■ Liberal Arts courses covered in secondary schools
		■ Transition is more seamless due to the exposure of courses and in some instances observations

TABLE 11.3 First-Year Curriculum: Accelerated Radiologic Science Programs

COURSE NAME	SEMESTER CREDIT HOURS
Fall Semester Year 1	
Anatomy and Physiology I	4
Algebra and Trigonometry	3
Expository Writing I	3
Introduction to Psychology	3
First-Year Seminar	1
Basic Chemistry I	4
Total	18
Spring Semester Year 1	
Anatomy and Physiology II	4
Physics	4
Expository Writing II	3
Computer Applications	3
Basic Chemistry II	4
Total	18

prerequisites prior to acceptance into the radiologic science associate degree programs. This translates into 3–4 years of college with the students being awarded an associate's degree.

MCPHS Accelerated Scheduling. MCPHS radiologic science majors are block scheduled, leaving the student a limited choice of electives. A further complication for accelerated students is the limited variety of liberal arts courses offered at a college that is solely focused on health professional studies. This results in the need to schedule electives at other colleges and universities associated within the collaborative network. The collaborative network, in our case, Colleges of the Fenway, is a consortium of six colleges: Wentworth Institute of Technology, Wheelock College, Simmons College, Massachusetts College of Art and Design, and Emmanuel College, centrally located in the Fenway area of Boston. These colleges offer a wide variety of majors not limited to the allied health field. The consortium allows students to take nonprofessional courses at any of these colleges.

The scheduling of core and professional course work is so rigid that time slots left available for elective courses are very limited. Time and traveling required for these classes infringe on the student's class and study time. Some class times of the collaborative institutions are not in sync with the MCPHS schedule. The students are required to leave courses early in order to arrive on time at another campus. They also may need to take these courses in the evenings. In some cases students may arrive home very late and are scheduled the following day for early classes or clinical.

If a student does not follow the requisite curriculum due to academic difficulties (e.g., failed course), the student will not finish the program in the allotted timeframe. These students are then out of the program sequence. An adjustment is required in the curriculum, changing their year of graduation. One solution is to have a nonaccelerated curriculum for those who request a more traditional college 4-year experience. One problem with this scenario is clinical space availability. Entry into the programs is based on allotment of clinical space. With multiple students moving their graduation year, difficulties arise with admission practices and accreditation requirements. Accrediting agencies clearly dictate student capacity for each clinical site.

The authors' perceived disadvantages of accelerated programs are that students may not have opportunities for extracurricular activities, for study-abroad experiences, or taking additional courses including independent research because of the course-laden schedule. Often, the selection of required electives is limited by the demands of professional coursework as stated earlier in the chapter. Table 11.4 identifies advantages and

TABLE 11.4 Advantages and Disadvantages of Accelerated Curricula: Comparison among The United States, Europe, and Australia

		UNITED STATES	EUROPE AND AUSTRALIA
Advantages		■ Cost ■ Retention in private colleges ■ Provide more students with educational opportunities, especially in the California state higher-education system ■ Decrease timeline for adult learners	■ Easier transition with a shorter interval between bachelors and masters ■ More mobility; students can move to other countries where the curriculum and length would be standardized ■ Transferring becomes almost seamless ■ Focused on more flexible learning pathways ■ Lifelong learning
Disadvantages		■ Compressed curriculum does not allow for full integration of college experience: abroad experiences, course selection limited, limited time available for part-time employment ■ Faculty have needed to schedule additional sections to meet the needs of the three programs	■ Mobility across other universities did not increase ■ Question of whether countries are internationally competitive ■ Course selection dictated more by scheduling than interest

disadvantages of accelerated curricula, with comparisons between the United States, Europe, and Australia.

ENROLLMENT AND DEMOGRAPHICS

Analysis of student data was used to determine any trends related to enrollments and demographics. To date, since the inception of the accelerated programs, 266 students have been enrolled, the average age being 19 years. Further analysis relating to the program's maximum and minimum ages are shown in Table 11.5. As demonstrated in the table, the school tends to attract more students from a younger demographic population, while the community colleges tend to attract an older population within the radiologic sciences. In comparison, a local community college with the largest enrollment in the radiologic sciences in the greater Boston area has a more mature student population. The average age is 27 (Bunker Hill Community College, 2010).

After implementing the 3-year accelerated degree program, the College did recognize changes in enrollments with increased student numbers in all three radiologic science programs, as shown in Table 11.6. The change to an accelerated format resulted in programs increasing the number of credit hours per semester and introducing summer session. This success prompted the College in adopting similar accelerated formats for the nursing, health sciences, and dental hygiene programs.

TABLE 11.5 Student Age Range MCPHS Radiologic Science Programs from 2002 to 2010

STUDENTS AGE (YEARS)	
Maximum	51
Minimum	17

TABLE 11.6 Change in Enrollments

	RADIATION THERAPY	RADIOGRAPHY	NUCLEAR MEDICINE TECHNOLOGY
Average 1998–2001	3.25	2.25	7.5
Average 2002–2007	12.7	14.8	13.2
% Change postaccelerated	390%	659%	176%
	Radiation therapy	Radiography	Nuclear medicine technology

LEARNING STRATEGIES

Technology

To support the student-centered learning and teaching philosophy, the college has several resources available. For example, Blackboard (educational platform) delivers content using nonnarrated and narrated Powerpoint lectures. Other popularly used web-based student response systems using Turning Technologies software and hardware include Articulate Presenter (narration software), Elluminate (virtual classroom), Google Apps, and Voicethread (video narration). These useful tools allow for additional online courses to be taught during traditional, early morning, and evening hours, giving flexibility to both students and faculty.

Pedagogy

Other techniques used in the classroom are games for review of content, critical thinking assignments, role playing, poster presentation, group projects, case study learning, Powerpoint presentations, clay modeling for anatomy, video modules to learn radiographic procedures, and student journaling. Students are required to verify their attendance at educational conferences organized by the clinical affiliates and professional societies. These conferences assist in developing personal networks for future job placement and help in contributing to lifelong learning skills.

FACULTY AND SUPPORT STAFF ROLES AND RESPONSIBILITIES

Of the total number of radiologic science students who have started the program, 75% have successfully completed the program in 3 years. Of these accelerated students, 47% are transfer students who come in with some prerequisites from community colleges or 4-year institutions. Students who enter the accelerated program with math and science GPAs of 2.5 or greater typically have a greater graduation rate. Before students are admitted into the school, open-house sessions run by the program faculty are provided to parents and prospective students with the potential curriculum, course load, and details on the accelerated schedule. Prospective students are encouraged to take advantage of the support services that the college provides as well as utilize course instructors for extra help. This procedure is again repeated during the early admission reception as well as the acceptance day open house.

During freshman orientation, students are divided into small breakout sessions based on their major. The radiologic science faculty meets with the students and reviews course load, progression standards, and pertinent information about each program. Students are once again reminded that if they begin to have trouble or feel that they need help with courses they should speak to their instructor or seek help at the Academic Resource center. All freshmen are required to take the course First Year Seminar 110. This course is designed to assist the student transitioning into college and balancing their time to create a healthy lifestyle. Peer mentors offer students a firsthand look at how to be successful by guiding and advising them based on their personal experiences.

The faculty advisor at the college monitors the student's progress in their first year to advocate early intervention where necessary. During the student's professional years, the program faculty oversees the student's performance in didactic courses and clinical internships. This is achieved by monitoring the grades throughout the semester and feedback from the adjunct professors. These students are given the option to convert to a 4-year program. Of these students who choose to do the programs in 4 years, 90% complete the program.

The Academic Resource Center functions to assist the student by providing academic advisors and counselors, disability support services, a writing center as well as a math center. The academic counselors meet with students and help them plan a strategy to become an effective, efficient individual learner. Peer tutors are available to work with student groups or on a one-to-one basis to assess student learning styles, set goals, and develop time management strategies.

The Writing Center assists the student in developing their writing skills, editing and proofreading skills, research, and improves vocabulary for developing a thesis, writing a summary, and so forth. The students are also supported psychologically by the counseling service. All information about these services is posted on the college website (MCPHS, 2011). Radiologic Science faculty members maintain an "open door policy" through email communication, face-to-face interactions, or personal tutoring. Faculties are required to post scheduled office hours as required by the college. These hours are included on class syllabi. The rigorous freshman courses are Anatomy and Physiology and Algebra and Trigonometry that contain 200 or more students in a lecture. These courses traditionally show the lowest number of students achieving a passing grade.

To address this issue, in 2010 the college divided the Anatomy & Physiology course into two sections, dividing the class size into half. Graduate students were hired to function as peer tutors for small-group tutoring sessions for those students who desired them. Also, the Adam software was made available to these students through the college library's website. With this software, students are able to review anatomy and physiology assignments, complete homework online, as well as test themselves utilizing the test bank independently. The last intervention is the early-warning system. Mid-semester, warning letters are sent to students notifying them of grades below passing, advising them to seek help to be successful in class.

The early intervention system has placed an added responsibility on the faculty. Teaching load has increased for instructors due to additional student resources. These interventions are implemented without the addition of more faculties. These early interventions have made a difference to the student who takes advantage of them. Many students who do not utilize these resources continue to struggle through their classes. If they are unsuccessful they do not advance into the next semester. To offer the students a smoother transition into college life, the faculties are looking to revamp the core curriculum by decreasing the total number of credits. In order to make these adjustments, some of the courses may be moved to summer sessions. We will be carefully monitoring this change to see whether the success of student learning and retention rates are improved.

FACULTY LIMITATIONS

The burden of this type of accelerated program rests heavily on the program faculty. Classes run throughout the year, with semester breaks reduced to accommodate two summer sessions as well as maintain 15-week spring and fall semesters. The break between spring and summer for the Radiation Therapy and Radiography Programs is reduced by 1 week to allow students more clinical time. The Nuclear Medicine Program conducts a 12-week summer session extending the normal summer session by 2 weeks. The faculty has limited time for research or professional development and vacation time in light of this full summer schedule of classes. Another challenge the faculties face is in trying to find the time to incorporate new technology tools, expand and improve course content, and revise accreditation standards.

FUTURE DIRECTIONS

Despite the limitations and challenges, the School of Radiologic Sciences has experienced growth in enrollments and the program model has been adopted across the institution for most undergraduate bachelors programs. To address some of the challenges posed by the compact format the faculty and adjuncts share some common courses such as Patient Care, Cross Sectional Anatomy, CT Imaging, Clinical Pathophysiology, Radiation Protection and Biology, and Medical Terminology. This coordination among the faculty addresses some of the challenges that face the School of Radiologic Sciences in using the accelerated format. This provides the basis for an interdisciplinary approach to educating the students to reflect current trends in clinical settings. Further developments focused on streamlining the curricula of the various programs and promoting the interdisciplinary approach are under discussion.

CONCLUSIONS

As the only college in the United States that offers an accelerated bachelors degree in the radiologic science disciplines, MCPHS provides a unique programmatic perspective. The programs have had a continued increase in enrollment due to a targeted marketing strategy, taking advantage of the attraction offered by the accelerated format. Graduates enter the work force at a faster rate than a traditional 4-year program graduate. These programs, however, put an increased strain on students due to higher course loads and the logistics of juggling the nonprofessional and professional course work with a clinical component. Students in these programs with the compressed curriculum do not have the advantage of balancing the academics with other school activities, giving them a less-than-well-rounded college experience seen as a rite of passage for most graduates.

We recognize the challenges and limitations of the accelerated format. Through ongoing discussion and continuing analysis of current trends we strive to create an environment of student success and assessment outcomes that meet or exceed our benchmarks. This can only be accomplished by collaborative efforts on the part of administration, faculty, and support services at the College.

REFERENCES

American Association of College of Nursing. (2010). *Accelerated programs: The fast-track to careers in nursing*. Retrieved from http://www.aacn.nche.edu/publications/issues/aug02.htm

Bunker Hill Community College. Retrieved from http://www.bhcc.mass.edu/inside/50

European Commission Education and Training. (2011). Retrieved from http://ec.europa.eu/education/higher-education/doc1290_en.htm

Health Career Center. (2011). Retrieved June 25, 2011 from http://www.healthcareer center.org/

Honan, W. (1993). Completing college in only 3 years? Idea is gaining support nation-wide. *The New York Times.* Retrieved from http://www.nytimes/1993/09/29/education/completing-college-in-only-3-years-idea-is

Massachusetts College of Pharmacy and Health Sciences. (2010). *College Catalogue 2010–2011.* Retrieved from http://www.mcphs.edu/academics/college_catalog/Massachusetts College of Pharmacy and Health Sciences

Morgan, J. Process Report Bologna lack a Coherent Europe-wide Focus. (2010). http://www.timeshighereducation.co.uk/story.asp?sectioncode=26&storycode=410886. Retrieved from http://www.mcphs.edu/academic_support_and_resources/index.html

Shellenbarger, S. (2010, May, 12). Speeding college to save $10,000. *The Wall Street Journal.* Retrieved from http://www.online.wsj.com/article/SB100014240 5274870356580452383341696523742.html

Wlodkowski, J. R., Mauldin, J. E., & Gahn, S. W. (2001). *Learning in the Fast Lane: Adult Learners' Persistence and Success in Accelerated College Programs*, 4(1), Lumina Foundation the Center for the Study of Accelerated Learning, School for Professional Studies, Regis University. Retrieved from http://www.luminafounda tion.org/publications/fastlane.pdf

Interprofessional Education: The Role of Accelerated Nursing Programs in Preparing the Nurse of the Future

*Paulette Seymour-Route, Janet Fraser Hale,
Michael Kneeland, and Michele Pugnaire*

INTRODUCTION

*"A*ll practice disciplines have specific teaching and learning challenges: learning in high stakes environments, confronting suffering and vulnerability; expertise depends on relational skills" (Benner, 2011, p. 224). Students entering the nursing profession today will be learning in an environment filled with challenges and opportunities. Traditional health care organizations have become more complex and are evolving into new health care delivery systems while adapting to the economic and reform-driven changes before us. Health care costs were estimated at $2.5 trillion in 2009 or 17.6% of the US gross domestic product (Martin, Lassman, Whittle, & Catlin, 2011) and costs are projected to grow as we address the access needs of the newly insured over the next few years. Quality and safety issues are a growing concern for many stakeholders; consumers, professionals, payers, and hospitals. A provider shortage continues to impede access to primary care and reform efforts. This includes a renewed focus on public health and health promotion. Preparing an adequate workforce of clinicians is hindered by the present and growing faculty shortage for nursing and other health professions

(Cronenwett & Dzau, 2010). However, the current environment provides the opportunity for innovation and change, stimulating all health care professionals to examine how we practice and how we teach.

The focus on patient-centered care unites all the practice professions. Interprofessional education (IPE), once a novel option, serves as a foundation to prepare nurses and other health professionals for the environment in which they will practice after graduation and into the future. The emphasis of this chapter lies on the opportunities that IPE holds for students and faculty in accelerated nursing programs. This chapter discusses the challenges, strategies, and ideas for integrating interprofessional learning into education programs for health professions. Specifically, the chapter focuses on IPE within accelerated nursing programs that are either second bachelor's, master's, or doctor of nursing practice as entry into the profession. The merits of and future for implementing IPE are addressed from the perspective of the impact on patient care, health care professionals, and the health care system.

BACKGROUND

Accelerated programs in nursing have been in place since 1971 (Beal, 2007) and nurse educators have had to address new ways of teaching and transitioning students into practice. The projected need to educate more professional and advanced practice nurses continues to be a challenge. Simultaneously, faculties are incorporating national recommendations for a better-educated nursing workforce. Accelerated programs are supported by the Joint Statement from the Tri-Council for Nursing (AACN, ANA, AONE, 2010) as an option to prepare the nurses needed to care for the aging baby boomers and people with acute and chronic illnesses. Additionally, nurses will need to respond to the call for public and community health services and health promotion activities for the population in the future. Primary, chronic, and acute care population needs can all benefit from team-based care (Reeves et al., 2009). Logically, IPE can support this patient-centered approach with the help of teams of providers.

INTERPROFESSIONAL EDUCATION

"Interprofessional Education (IPE) occurs when two or more professions learn with, from and about each other to improve collaboration and the quality of care" (CAIPE, 2002, p. 224).

IPE includes a wide range of learning opportunities. Before a program begins the process of designing IP educational activities, agreement on mutual goals must be reached among all interprofessional partners. Core competencies for health professionals can include communication, collaboration, professionalism, and teamwork. Current health professional curricula may need to be redesigned to facilitate the learning goals and competencies that support IPE. Therefore, each IPE program partnership may select different opportunities and/or a different timeline.

Currently, many health profession educators believe that team-based care provides the best approach to practice safe, high-quality patient care (Macy, 2010 Conference Summary). Health professions should learn together with a full understanding of each other's roles, priorities, expertise, and experience. Team-based learning is the ideal model, given that it immediately and inherently demonstrates the skills and expertise of each of the professions resulting in coordinated care. Health profession education has common core basic foundational components such as anatomy, physiology, biochemistry, pathology, pharmacology, assessment, communication skills, the patient—provider relationship, crisis management, ethics, health policy, population health, legal issues in health care, research methods, evaluation of literature, and evidence-based practice. Teaching these basics simultaneously to students from multiple disciplines while drawing on faculty expertise from a variety of professions is an opportunity for not only the delivery of the content, but also collaborating for the evaluation of both the learners and the effect of IPE on health care outcomes.

A deep insight into the history of IPE informs the challenges and opportunities present today. Interest in interprofessional learning can be traced back to more than 50 years (Szasz, 1969). Increased emphasis began in the 1970s with a surge in the literature in the 1990s (Atkins & Walsh, 1997; Barr, 1998; Barrington et al., 1998; Harris, Starnaman, Henry, & Bland, 1998) and continuing to the present (Cooke, Irby, & O'Brien, 2010; IOM, 2010; Miller, Moore, Stead, & Balser, 2010). Interprofessional health professions education began in community clinics in the 1960s with the development of Neighborhood Health Centers providing care to indigent populations. In the 1980s, the U.S. Veterans Administration initiated interprofessional geriatric treatment teams to care for aging veterans. In 1993, President Clinton initiated health care reform initiatives, focusing on managing health care costs, increasing access to care, and improving the quality of health care. These initiatives seeded the movement that continues to forge changes in health care delivery and health care provider roles and practice patterns in the United States today.

National accrediting organizations for nursing and medicine began to address IPE in the 1990s. In 1995, The Association of American Medical Colleges (AAMC) and Liaison Committee on Medical Education (LCME) recommended interdisciplinary courses as one of the means for increasing communication and collaboration among members of the health professions (AAMC, 1995). The American Association of Colleges of Nursing (AACN) published a *Position Statement on Interdisciplinary Education and Practice* that promotes collaboration as emanating from an understanding and appreciation of the roles and contributions that each discipline brings to the care delivery system, resulting from shared educational and practice experiences (AACN, 1996), and continues in the AACN white paper on the role of the Clinical Nurse Leader (AACN, 2007) and the AACN Essentials for the Doctor of Nursing Practice (AACN, 2006). Across all levels of nursing practice programs, IPE is recognized as an important learning activity contributing to successful practice and relevant to patient outcomes. Over the years, since the 1970s, terms referring to IPE include interdisciplinary, collaborative, and team-based (Macy, 2010 Conference Summary) and will be used interchangeably.

How did the focus on IPE gain the momentum it enjoys today in health professions education in the United States? There are probably many answers, but none more important than the impact of the quality and safety movement. The Institute for Medicine (IOM) Quality of Health Care in America Committee was established in 1998 (IOM, 2000) and set the strategic direction for health professions that continue today. The report *To Err is Human: Building a Safer Health System*, released in 1999 and published in 2000, includes a recommendation for health care organizations and affiliated professionals to develop patient safety programs that included the establishment of *interdisciplinary team* training programs that incorporate proven methods of team training, such as simulation (IOM, 2000). The focus on team training has been enhanced and demonstrated improved quality and safety for hospital patients (Baker, Gustafson, Beaubien, Salas, & Barach, 2005). The notion of lifelong learning as a competency and ongoing education in teams for physicians and nurses has been developed by the AAMC and AACN with support from the Macy Foundation (AACN/AAMC, 2010).

The IOM promotes the need for IPE and collaboration through a series of reports (IOM, 2000, 2001, 2003). *Crossing the Quality Chasm* documented disturbing shortfalls in the quality of health care in the United States, including the system changes needed to decrease the sizable gap between what we know from evidence and what we do in clinical practice (IOM, 2001). *Health Professions Education: A Bridge to Quality* made recommendations on the education of health professional competencies including: all health professionals to be educated to deliver patient-centered care as members of an interdisciplinary team with emphasis on evidence-based practice, quality improvement, and informatics (IOM, 2003). These reports consistently call for health care providers to work together with a collective sense of accountability for patient and health outcomes. These policy reports demonstrate a paradigm shift in health care delivery away from individual providers toward teams of providers focusing on outcomes of care for the individuals and populations served (IOM, 2003). This paradigm shift has an impact on every health care setting.

CURRENT NATIONAL PERSPECTIVE: IPE

Over the past two years, the emphasis on curriculum reform for nurses and physicians has received significant attention from the Carnegie Foundation (Benner, Sutphen, Leonard, & Day, 2010; Cooke et al., 2010). *Educating nurses: A call for radical transformation* presents the nursing community with recommendations that will transform the educational process with the intent of preparing well-educated nurses. Point-of-care teaching, practice in teams, and an accelerated educational approach are among the recommended changes to produce the kind and number of nurses needed now and in the future (Benner et al., 2010). The Carnegie report *Educating Physicians: A call for reform of medical school and residency* has also addressed the changes needed in schools of medicine to meet patient care needs (Cooke et al., 2010). The scope, magnitude, and timeliness of the transformational change are exciting and the implementation will be challenging. Positive gains for patient-centered care and provider satisfaction will be realized if we can maintain the distinct contribution of each discipline while practicing in teams of lifelong learners.

The Institute of Medicine (IOM) Robert Wood Johnson (RWJ) *Future of Nursing: Leading Change, Advancing Health* report released in October 2010 takes the agenda even further (IOM, 2010). This report addresses the need for action by all health care providers to act now to remodel the health care system. The report recommends that nurses be full partners with physicians and others in redesigning the US health care system. The report calls for more nurses in the workforce at the baccalaureate level or higher by 2020. The role of new and innovative curricular models for educating our future nurses is recommended.

The role of IPE seems clear, important, and supported by national initiatives. IPE requires students, faculty, and all health professionals to work together to share teaching and learning environments for increased collaboration, partnerships, and team building. Despite the importance of IPE, implementation has been slow as noted by Chow (2011), "the future is here, it just isn't everywhere." Changes in science, technology, policy, and systems are the new norm. Our approaches to educating the practice professions need to evolve and keep pace! Understanding the challenges may help to guide the development of strategies and future direction for IPE.

CHALLENGES TO IPE

Any new initiative or proposed change to the status quo may be perceived as threatening to those who may be affected by the change. Introduction of a new paradigm often results in both subtle and not-so-subtle resistance. Inevitably, a change of the magnitude that IPE represents will stress resources and generate debate about whether or not it should be done. Miller et al. (2010) describe the change needed in health professions education as a disruptive innovation. Common challenges follow.

Disciplinary Silos

At many institutions, professional schools are separate, each with their own "building(s)" with duplicity of educational space, some courses, faculty of various sub-disciplines, and separate and distinct clinical experiences. School-specific schedules are also challenging. The various health professional schools in any given university or academic health science center may have different academic terms with different length semesters—including start and end dates, timing, sequencing, and leveling of courses in their respective curricula, including restrictive parameters for numbers of students who can enroll. Physical space limitations (classroom size and numbers available) may prohibit larger classes consisting of students from other disciplines. Lack of small group meeting rooms may preclude small group interprofessional gatherings and initiatives. Lastly, and perhaps most challenging, is the belief of the purists, who will argue that the real world of their discipline is such that IPE would not withstand the true academic rigor required by their profession. Within the "silos" are the specific requirements of the professional and academic accrediting bodies that have historically been slow to include standards that would support major interprofessional initiatives (Miller et al., 2010).

Current Reward and Recognition Processes

It is important to recognize the invisible nature of the time and effort that goes into creating successful interprofessional learning opportunities. Historically, this has been one of the strongest countervailing forces in most institutions. This invisibility contributes to the current status of negligible tangible faculty reward or recognition for interprofessional efforts. For the most part, promotion and tenure decisions are largely based on rewarding faculty for their research productivity. Teaching and service (predominantly referring to university service) may be viewed as necessary, but rarely sufficient, for serious consideration for promotion and tenure. The efforts and initiatives for interdisciplinary courses and IPE community-service learning may be perceived as "soft," taking valuable time away from more important classes and clinical time specific to their discipline, and/or as a distraction from their perceived mandates for promotion within their institution, or other professional and regulatory requirements. This perception is slowly beginning to change as more national publications and health care reform briefs support the importance of IPE.

Student Characteristics

Another debate surrounding IPE initiatives is the belief that students of various professions are at different developmental stages in terms of age, experience, maturity, professional expectations, attitudes, and intellect. These perceived differences are believed to preclude common course work and common approaches to education. For example, medical students are generally in their early 20s, recently out of undergraduate education, or with one to two years of research, service, or work experience, while Physician Assistant (PA) students and Nurse Practitioner (NP) students are usually older, with a number of years of health care experience. The generic entry-level nursing students may be recent high-school graduates and can be from a number of academic entry points into nursing, that is, diploma, associate's degree, or entry-level baccalaureate. These concerns are less likely to be present in accelerated programs. Like medical students, dental students, and physical therapy students, applicants for accelerated programs [whether they are students in second bachelor's, master's, or doctor of nursing practice (DNP) programs] have successfully completed a baccalaureate degree, and similar to medical school applicants, may have spent a couple of years in research, national or international public service, or in another profession. Accelerated nursing students may be the most appropriate nursing students to participate with all the other graduate professional entry programs in IPE activities as they are similar, in terms of age and stage of intellectual development, to students who apply to medical and other postbaccalaureate health professions' schools. Their acceptance into accelerated nursing programs is equally competitive, as they are competing with many other highly qualified individuals for the limited space in accelerated programs (AACN Fact Sheet, 2010a; AACN Issue Bulletin, 2010b). Most accelerated programs follow schedules more like other graduate-level health professions schools. Students are likely to be on campus for courses or in clinical or lab settings five days a week, eight hours a day. Joint social as well as academic programming can easily be planned based on students' increased presence on campus for at least the first year or two of their postbaccalaureate education. Their academic programming includes didactic coursework and interprofessional case-based clinical and simulation exercises. These types of exercises provide an excellent forum for joint problem-solving by health professions students early in their programs of study. Early academic introduction to health care concepts and experiences for students in IPE are key to building future interdisciplinary relationships through early collaboration and the development of trust necessary to provide team-based care in the future.

Implications of IPE: Resources, Budgets, Promotion, and Tenure

Funding of schools within universities and colleges varies. A school may receive an allocation from the university or school within a college or university based on the revenue they generate as a school from tuition, fees, or other service arrangements. Faculty are generally hired by a specific school and workloads are generated by each school to meet the specific needs of that school to achieve their mission. The models for faculty in a school of nursing may differ significantly from that of a school of medicine, especially for schools attached to an academic health science center where faculty are practicing clinicians. These differences contribute to the challenge of equitable compensation and workload for those involved in IPE across disciplines. Success requires significant trust, collaboration, and support from all involved in school/programs and their leadership. Grants and start-up funding may be available initially, but resources to sustain the program need to be addressed within the IPE implementation plan.

In summary, the challenges for IPE are many, but not insurmountable. The logistics can be overwhelming for those without the will, passion, and perseverance to make it happen. A champion from each discipline is essential. Successful IPE programs will require: dedicated faculty, manageable workloads, faculty development, and technology. Equally important will be visible demonstration of the value and the recognition of these efforts by the university/college through: recognition of IPE as important for promotion and tenure, infrastructure support, and adequate resources to evaluate and sustain the IP effort over time. IPE needs solid commitment from leadership, faculty committed to the concept, students who value the IPE learning experience, and health care consumers who see the benefit of team-based care. Table 12.1 provides a summary of challenges for IPE.

TABLE 12.1   Challenges for Interprofessional Education

GENERAL CHALLENGE	DETAILS
Disciplinary silos	■ Isolation of schools goes well beyond merely the proximity of professional schools from each other: For example, different academic calendars, tuition rates, credit allocation, semester schedules and limited. ■ If common coursework is combined, faculty may lose positions. ■ IP education will result in the loss of the academic rigor required of respective disciplines.
Current reward and recognition processes for faculty	■ IPE efforts invisible and not (or less) valued than the more traditional views of teaching, practice, and research/scholarship for promotion and tenure. ■ Contributions/teaching of students outside of the discipline is "invisible," not valued, and perceived as not helping the school mission. ■ Workloads rarely include IPE since it does not support school-specific mission.
Student characteristics	■ Students are perceived as dissimilar. (Multiple levels of entry into basic nursing practice). ■ Accelerated nursing students offer a more similar highly competitive student profile and are more similar to those of other health professions entry programs.
Resource and budgetary implications	■ Historically, resources and budgets are allocated strictly by and to each professional school to meet their respective missions.
IPE is not yet included in the discipline specific standards for accreditation by national accrediting organizations	■ While they are all beginning to espouse it, it is not yet evident in any of the significant evaluation components for accreditation, and thus the absolute impetus to conform to the expectation is not in place.

EVIDENCE SUPPORTING INTERPROFESSIONAL LEARNING

Cooper, Carlisle, Gibbs, and Watkins (2001) published a systematic review on the evidence base for interdisciplinary learning in undergraduate education. The authors recognized the need to examine the traditional processes used for a systematic review and adapted their methodology to include educational evaluation and outcomes literature, and qualitative as well as quantitative research. The review noted a lack of theoretical or conceptual underpinnings for the studies reviewed. Points of interest relevant to IPE for accelerated nursing students include: (1) early learning experiences resulted in future participation in interdisciplinary activities, (2) the importance of students being at a similar stage of intellectual development for maximal benefit, (3) support and role modeling from a consistent team of faculty and administrators as conducive to positive outcomes, (4) problem-based learning, and (5) understanding and respecting the role of each discipline associated with the experience.

IPE Readiness

Thannhauser, Russell, Mayhew, and Scott (2010) reviewed the interprofessional literature for instruments used to measure engagement in IPE and collaboration. Two are of particular interest: the Readiness for Interprofessional Learning Scale and the Interdisciplinary Perception Scale developed by Luecht Madsen, Taugher, and Petterson (1990). McFadyen et al. (2005) published results of their content analysis of the Readiness for Interprofessional Learning Scale originally published by Parsell and Bligh (1999). The nineteen-question scale has been used in the United Kingdom and seems to be promising as a measure to evaluate IPE interventions. At the Centre for Excellence in Interprofessional Education in Belfast, Morison, Johnston, and Stevenson (2010) have developed the Studying and Learning Preferences Inventory (SALPI) to determine student readiness for IPE (McFadye et al., 2005). Accelerated nursing programs with IPE activities may consider using such instruments to measure students' readiness for IPE.

IPE: The Educator

A review by Reeves et al. (2009) evaluated the effect of IPE on health professionals and found that improvement was demonstrated in how professionals worked together and in the care the patients received.

Zwarenstein, Goldman, and Reeves (2009) built upon the work with a subsequent systematic review, *Interprofessional collaboration: Effects of practice-based interventions on professional practice and healthcare outcomes.* The small number ($n = 5$) of studies included one or more of the following types of collaboration: interprofessional rounds, meetings, or audits with mixed results. It is clear that more rigorous studies are needed to provide evidence in support of IPE and its impact on patient health outcomes.

Teams

Baker and colleagues (2005) prepared a report to the Agency for Heathcare Research and Quality (AHRQ) titled *Medical teamwork and patient safety: The evidence-based relation.* The report includes training models and strategies relevant to IPE and examines the science of team performance and team training research relevant to medical teams, patient safety, and error reduction. Accelerated nursing programs and their IP partners can reference this report for designing IPE curriculum and activities. Sarani et al. (2009) examined the perceptions of residents and RNs of the impact of a medical emergency team on education and patient safety. Although the survey was conducted in a single site, the results were encouraging. Both groups believed that the team improved patient safety without compromising the educational experience.

Continuous Learning Model

Miller et al. (2010) emphasized the consensus of the national experts to craft a new vision of a health care workforce comprised of physicians and other professionals, all of whom are capable of assessing practice outcomes, identifying learning needs, and engaging in continuous learning to achieve the best care for their patients. The training for this model should start at the beginning of the education process leading to true IPE, with shared facilities and the same basic coursework (Miller et al., 2010). The authors revisit the Flexner report on medical education published in 1910 and make significant recommendations for a model and approach to the education of the health care workforce. Their approach is comprehensive and innovative. The authors fittingly describe their approach as a "disruptive technology". The underlying principles for the model come from a Vanderbilt University School of Medicine proposal for medical education reform. The underlying principles include: (1) learning is competency based and imbedded in the workplace, (2) all workers learn; all learners work, (3) learning is undertaken by individuals, teams, and institutions and is linked to patient needs, (4) learning activities are modular; the system allows multiple entry and exit points, (5) learning is interprofessional, with shared facilities, common schedules, and shared foundational coursework, (6) a rich technology infrastructure supports the health care learning system and (7) health outcomes and educational outcomes are directly linked. The principles proposed in this model are aligned with an efficient approach across all accelerated programs in nursing and with various recommendations from the Carnegie Foundation (Benner et al., 2010; Cooke et al., 2010; Miller et al., 2010, p. 267) and the Josiah Macy Foundation (2010). These principles also support lifelong learning that is essential for baccalaureate and graduate nursing students.

In summary, the movement toward IPE is growing, including efforts to further develop valid evaluation and measurement for IPE interventions and outcomes. Whatever model, framework, or point on the IPE continuum an accelerated nursing program chooses as a starting point, it is essential to determine the relevant competencies. The following section discusses the more common competencies associated with IPE.

COMPETENCIES

Health Professions Education: A Bridge to Quality promotes five core competencies that all clinicians should possess, regardless of their discipline, to meet the needs of the 21st-century health system. These core competencies include: (1) provide patient-centered care, (2) work in interdisciplinary teams, (3) employ evidence-based practice, (4) apply quality improvement principles, and (5) utilize informatics (IOM, 2003). In support of the national initiative from the IOM (2003), the Quality and Safety Education for Nurses (QSEN) project has focused on developing the knowledge, skills, and attitudes (KSAs) for educating nurses in patient-centered care, teamwork and collaboration, evidence-based practice, quality improvement, safety, and informatics for both professional and advanced practice nurses (2011). The KSAs can serve accelerated professional nursing and IPE programs with competency-specific information that is useful for curriculum development.

The Massachusetts Nursing Initiative (2010), through the Nurse of the Future Committee, has developed a series of competencies for the professional nurse. Building upon the IOM (2003) and QSEN (2011) competencies, the project includes other related competencies:

professionalism, system-based practice, and communication at the level necessary to enter practice as a professional nurse. Accelerated nursing programs can benefit from the specificity of the KSAs for entry into practice from the model and address IPE opportunities for professional nursing students.

The Interprofessional Education Collaborative (IPEC), a partnership of six national education associations of health professions, including nursing, medicine, pharmacy, dentists, osteopathic medicine, and public health formed in 2009 to promote IPE. IPEC has recently released two reports. First developed is a set of core competencies for interprofessional collaborative practice. Table 12.2 includes the four core competency domains with further explanation/summary competency statement for each domain (IPEC, 2011a). These core competencies can be integrated into the curriculum of accelerated programs and serve as a foundation for designing and evaluating joint learning activities.

Health Resources and Services Administration (HRSA) convened a 2011 conference titled *Team-Based Competencies: Building a Shared Foundation for Education and Clinical Practice* in partnership with

TABLE 12.2   Core Competences for Interprofessional Collaborative Practice

INTERPROFESSIONAL COMPETENCY DOMAINS	EXPLANATION
Values/Ethics for interprofessional practice	Work with individuals of other professions to maintain a climate of mutual respect and shared values
Roles/Responsibilities for collaborative practice	Use the knowledge of one's own role and the roles of other professions to appropriately assess and address the health care needs of the patients and populations served
Interprofessional communication	Communicate with patients, families, communities, and other health professionals in a responsive and responsible manner that supports a team approach to maintaining health and treatment of disease
Interprofessional teamwork and team-based care	Apply relationship-building values and the principles of team dynamics to perform effectively in different team roles to plan and deliver patient/population-centered care that is safe, timely, efficient, effective, and equitable Other areas for future focus
IPE evaluation research	Opportunities include outcomes of student learning, application, quality, safety, and patient/population outcomes of team-based care
Increased dissemination of Best Practices for IPE	Publications and presentations at national conferences of what universities and colleges are doing in support of IPE
Further dissemination of effective strategies to overcome the challenges	Each college/university is unique and creative approaches to overcome the challenges should be shared through publication and presentations

the Macy Foundation, the Robert Wood Johnson Foundation (RWJF), and the American Board of Internal Medicine (ABIM) Foundation with the IPEC. Eighty academic and clinical leaders from around the country were invited to review the 2011 IPEC *Core Competencies for Interprofessional Collaborative Practice* to develop action plans for the implementation of these competencies into education and health care delivery. This second publication identified five action strategies: (1) communicate and disseminate, (2) develop interprofessional faculty and resources, (3) strengthen metrics and research, (4) develop new collaborative academic practices and new collaborations with community learning sites, and (5) advance policy changes (IPEC, 2011b). See Table 12.2 for the core competences for interprofessional collaborative practice.

STRATEGIES: EXEMPLARS OF CURRENT AND FUTURE INTERPROFESSIONAL INITIATIVES

The purpose of this section is to (1) generate new ideas or refine current IP initiatives for accelerated programs already embarking on IPE and (2) to spark interest toward possible initiatives for accelerated programs that may not have considered IPE opportunities. An overview of large national IPE initiatives, previously and currently sponsored by the Josiah Macy, Jr. Foundation, are presented. Exemplars of initiatives are briefly described regarding the planning, implementation, and subsequent evaluation stages. Each exemplar addresses efforts used to overcome challenges and barriers such as disciplinary silos, professional cultures and socialization, lack of multiple health professions schools at an institution, the importance of communication and teamwork, the need for faculty development to move beyond the status quo, and the importance of outside funding to support some of the initial resourcing issues with IP efforts.

The Macy Foundation has been funding health care initiatives since 1930 and is the only national foundation "devoted solely to improving the education of health professionals" (Josiah Macy Foundation, 2010, p. 21). The Foundation President George Thibault reports that the Foundation currently serves as a participant in the discussions on the role of health professions education in the context of health care reform. Macy funding is focused "at the intersection of health professions education and health care delivery" (Josiah Macy, 2010, pp. 6–7). In June 2010, the Foundation cohosted a conference with the Carnegie Foundation for the Advancement of Teaching to advance new models for IPE in academic health centers. The conference brought together Deans and other leaders of medical and nursing schools from seven academic health science centers. The major themes from this conference include: (1) determining optimal content and timing for IPE, (2) overcoming logistical barriers inherent in efforts to train students from different schools together, (3) providing faculty with opportunities to develop interprofessional teaching skills, (4) creating better evaluation and measurement tools, and (5) developing a team identity alongside specific professional identity (Josiah Macy Foundation, 2010, p. 15).

The prelude to the 2010 funding was a previous Josiah Macy, Jr. Foundation IPE initiative that identified the following strategies to overcome some of the challenges (Josiah Macy Foundation, 2010, p. 17). These were: (1) the logistical reasons for not doing IPE can be overcome with good leadership support from the top, (2) IP initiatives must be rigorous with clear educational objectives and metrics, and (3) the greatest impact is accomplished by repeated IP experiences occurring over time and in a variety of settings.

The Josiah Macy, Jr. Foundation grants supporting IPE may be germane to accelerated nursing programs. The University of Colorado Denver, for example, designed their new medical complex specifically to facilitate and integrate IPE. They plan to fully integrate the commonalities of curricula for all the schools on campus (medicine, nursing, physician assistant, physical therapy, dentistry, and pharmacy) to help students gain competencies in teamwork, collaborative care, quality, and safety. This curriculum will span the students' educational experience and facilitate interaction throughout their curricula. Students begin with a health mentors program that is built on a series of patient-centered tasks and integrated basic science, clinical care, and prevention with social and behavioral sciences and team-based skill building. Interprofessional student groups will be matched with families, including a patient with chronic illness who are living in the community. These IPE experiences will span throughout the early few years of students' learning. In the more highly focused clinical years, they plan to integrate a clinical communication tool for students to use in simulation exercises of complex patient issues. Residents and faculty will be involved, as well, through faculty development initiatives promoting the IPE concept and practice beyond core educational experiences (Macy, 2010b).

Case Western Reserve has been funded to develop and implement a multi-disciplinary curriculum that will incorporate collaborative learning experiences, real-life learning labs, and development of a virtual center supporting ongoing faculty and curricular development. Their plans include multidiscipline student teams working in acute care, as well as in a student-run free community clinic to further hone their team-building skills (Josiah Macy Foundation Grantees, 2010a).

Vanderbilt University has partnered its medical and nursing schools with health professions schools from three other universities bringing in social work and pharmacy students. They plan to implement this initiative as a pilot program through the *Fellowship in IP Learning*. Their goal is to ensure that students achieve the competencies to deliver the highest quality and safest care to their patients. Their approach is based on the assumption that a cultural change is needed to move beyond the current social and cultural assumptions within the individual professional school, specifically, and overcome the very challenging but "seemingly mundane issues" such as the coordination of schedules and calendars (Josiah Macy Foundation Grantees, 2010c, pp. 27–28). Their model addresses early IP experiences before the assimilation of cultural assumptions of their individual professions; and that "logistical obstacles can be overcome by institutional will" (Josiah Macy Foundation Grantees, 2010c, pp. 27–28). Their proposal is based on a number of principles, including that learning should be competency based, learning outcomes and healthcare outcomes will be directly linked when learning is situated in the healthcare delivery environment, and, lastly, health professionals should be trained in the IP model from the outset of their educational processes (Josiah Macy Foundation Grantees, 2010c).

The Weill Cornell Medical College and Hunter College are funded to provide students with an understanding of the value and contributions of different professional identities. They will enhance collaborative behavior using Giltell's theory of relational coordination as the organizing framework to develop curriculum. The theory is defined as "a mutually reinforcing process of interaction between communication and relationships carried out for the purpose of task integration." Unique to this theory is the fact that it emphasizes how communication among team members is frequent, timely, accurate, and effective. Communication is based on mutual respect, shared knowledge, and shared goals, and focuses on problem solving (Josiah Macy Foundation Grantees, 2010d, pp. 27–28; Giltell, 2002, pp. 1408–1426).

In 2006, the University of Minnesota initiated the requirement for all health professions students to meet collaborative competencies in professionalism and ethics, communication, and teamwork (Josiah Macy Conference Summary, 2010). The University of New Mexico's recent initiative is the development of an interprofessional experience for health professions students, law students, and community partners to prepare students to address issues of domestic violence. An earlier pilot of the program demonstrated outcomes that increased student knowledge of community resources for victims and families experiencing domestic violence, as well as small group interprofessional plans to help families reduce their risk of recurring violence (Josiah Macy Conference Summary, 2010).

It is anticipated that the findings from each of these studies, along with others not discussed, will provide a national roadmap for dissemination, expansion, and enhancement of IPE. In terms of challenges to overcome, they emphasized the importance of support from senior leadership, early integration of IP learning in the professions' educational programs, and working in real-life settings for team building and problem-solving.

In Spring 2011, the Josiah Macy, Jr. Foundation's *New Integrated Interprofessional Curriculum Model* in partnership with the Institute on Medicine as a Profession funded five academic institutions, including the University of Massachusetts Worcester (UMW) to participate in the *Education and Training to Professionalism*. The UMW interprofessional curriculum will focus on developing and promoting professionalism and patient-centered care within small groups of students for integration across schools, disciplines, and specialties. This curriculum will build on existing medical and graduate nursing curricula [focusing on students from the Graduate Entry Pathway (GEP)] in professionalism, ethics, and IPE.

One of eight academic health science centers recently selected by the Carl J. Shapiro Institute for Education and Research of Harvard University and the Macy Foundation, UMW medical, graduate nursing, and education faculty participated at a national invitational meeting focused on teaching critical thinking in interdisciplinary models at the 2011 Millennium Conference. The conference focused faculty from three disciplines to work together to develop curricular innovations in critical thinking, using interprofessional approaches that span the health sciences and the continuum of learners: from student to resident to practicing professional. Moving curricula beyond passive didactics to more interaction between and among the IP learners and faculty was emphasized. Table 12.3 describes strategies for successful intervention of IPE.

EXEMPLARS OF SUSTAINED AND ONGOING INITIATIVES

George Mason University/George Washington University IP Initiatives

In 1986, an IP initiative led by two visionary national nursing leaders, Dr. Doreen Harper then at George Mason University (GMU) College of Nursing and Health Science (public institution in Northern Virginia) and Dr. Jean Johnson at The George Washington University (GWU) School of

TABLE 12.3   Strategies for Successful Intervention of Interprofessional Education

ESSENTIAL STRATEGY	RATIONALE
Support from senior institutional leadership with a "champion" in each of the participating professional schools is essential	The logistical challenges can be overcome with good leadership support from the top. No sense in pursuing until this is present
Faculty from each school dedicated to the IP initiative	These are the folks who can make it happen in their courses and classes. Won't happen without their support
Schools must provide for flexibility in schedules, academic calendars	All schools will need to compromise and be open to scheduling changes. It is okay for different programs within schools to have different semester start and end dates as long as they fall within a broad school semester schedule
Integrate the commonalities of curricula among the professions to decrease duplication of efforts	This may pose a threat to content-specific faculty in each school (fear of loss of position), but is an essential area to develop efficiency and common ground in IP education
Early integration of IP learning in the professions' educational programs. Curriculum should span the students' educational experience and facilitate interaction throughout their curricula	The greatest impact is accomplished by early onset and repeated IP experiences occurring over time and in a variety of settings: inpatient, outpatient, long-term care, and community
Incorporate highly interactive case-based and clinical/community-based IP learning	Generates interest among students to collectively problem-solve for optimal patient care regardless of setting
Working in simulated and real-life settings for team building and problem-solving.	Creates the environment for what they will face when in practice
Develop a team identity alongside specific professional identity	This is part of the sea change in culture. Would not be easy to break down territorial barriers for solely professional identity
IP initiatives must be rigorous with clear educational objectives and metrics and	Early IP experiences before the assimilation of cultural assumptions of their individual professions and trained in the IP model from the outset of their educational experiences; and that "logistical obstacles can be overcome by institutional will"
Review appointment, promotion, and tenure documents to ensure valuation of IP education/teaching/clinical/research for promotion and tenure	Place increased emphasis and workload allocation for faculty who embrace IPE in recognition for promotion and tenure criteria

(Continued)

TABLE 12.3 Continued

ESSENTIAL STRATEGY	RATIONALE
Build in evaluation components in university IPE plan. Evaluate outcomes of student learning c/w graduate competencies and in terms of patient and population outcomes	There is a dearth of evidence in support for the actual outcomes and impact of IPE
Provide faculty with opportunities to develop interprofessional teaching skills	Faculty and resident faculty development is essential for sustaining and for the inculcation of lifelong learning. Faculty development is essential for them to learn the best approaches to IPE; some of these skills are not intuitive
Create evaluation and measurement tools	Several have been discussed in this article

Medicine and Health Sciences (private institution) in the District of Columbia, partnered to begin a collaborative nurse practitioner program at GMU. GMU collaborated with the leadership of the long-established GWU medical school and physician assistant program for selected common coursework. In 1995, the two universities developed another interprofessional initiative known as the Interdisicplinary Student Community Oriented Prevention Services (ISCOPES) program, which incorporated five health disciplines (graduate nursing students from GMU and medical, physician assistant, public health, physical therapy, and health systems management students from GWU) in community service-learning initiatives to support poorly resourced communities to promote health for the underserved populations in Washington, DC and Northern Virginia. This initiative has continually expanded over the years through student dedication of the leadership. The ongoing interprofessional presence in these underserved communities has made significant contributions to the health and well-being of populations in DC and VA. The authors cite these two IPE initiatives, in particular, as an example of how a nursing program at a traditional university can partner successfully with an academic health science center from another major university. Both the collaborative NP Program and the ISCOPES programs overcame all the challenges described earlier, along with a few more. For example, they forged a partnership between a public and private institution that spans state lines, schools, and universities with very different missions, schedules, and tuition rates. The GMU/GWU initiatives have endured for over two decades.

UMass Worcester IP Initiative

IP initiatives at UMass Worcester (UMW) date back to the early 1990s. Early partnerships started and continue with joint voluntary activities, such as providing care at free clinics in the community and joint academic initiatives such as interclerkships (half- to one-day foci on topics of interest) and mini-selectives (small groups of graduate nursing students and fourth-year medical students who are immersed in intensive week-long exposure to various specialties). Both interclerkships and mini-selectives involve expert speakers, small group work, case-based discussions, and joint clinical opportunities. Examples of interclerkship and mini-selective interest areas include oral health, women's health, violence and abuse, elder care services, end-of-life care, and palliative care. In addition, optional enrichment electives open to medical, graduate nursing students, and recently including pharmacy students from a neighboring school are available each year to interested students. Examples of these IP classes are Medical Interviewing in Spanish, The US Health Care System, Health Policy, Rural Health Scholars, Adoption and Foster Care and a Geriatric Patient Navigator Program.

Similar to the GMU/GWU ISCOPES program, UMW requires all medical and accelerated pathway graduate nursing students to participate in a community service-learning experience with vulnerable populations and medically underserved communities as part of a Population Health Clerkship (PHC). IP clerkship groups are based full time (80 hours over two weeks) in their respective communities. Each group is led by two faculty coleaders from different disciplines, schools, and/or community sites. In 2009, dental residents and pharmacy students began to participate in selected PHC groups as well. The Population Health Clerkship is based on an ecological framework of the multiple determinants of health and well-being for patients, families, and communities. Specifically, during each fall following the prelicensure year, GEP students in the community health component of their degree and medical students in the second basic science year prioritize their choices for a community placement. The options range from teams in free health care clinics, homeless shelters, elder services, to correctional health facilities. Working together in teams on these projects, the students gain insight into the strengths of both professions in an environment some call a "community of practice." Drawing on the expertise of each of the professions, they complete the course requirements including a comprehensive population health framework, jointly determining an identified need specific to their community, both of which inform a group poster session for the university community at large at the end of the clerkship.

Following the clerkship, all the GEP students (required) and some of the other health professions' students (voluntary) continue in their respective settings for an additional 45 or more hours to further implement and evaluate needed programming or interventions identified during the Population Health Clerkship. Many excellent deliverables have resulted from these initiatives. For example, one group working on an obesity prevention program for a rural elementary school submitted a proposal and received a $50,000 grant to implement and sustain their program.

Registered nurse graduate students teaching technical skills to medical students has been a project developed over many years now, at UMW. In this model, graduate nursing and medical students work together each fall to plan and implement influenza clinics for the local medically underserved populations. Prior to the flu clinic offerings, the GSN students hold two, two-hour classes, formally instructing the medical students on *Best Practices for Administering Injections*. In 2006, with the opening of the new UMW Simulation Center this initiative expanded to include a pilot program for *Best Practices for IV Insertion*. The IV classes were well received by both the graduate nursing student "teachers" and the medical student "learners." After the first pilot offering, it was quickly institutionalized into each block of the 12-week *Surgical Clerkship* to reach all third-year medical students over the course of the year.

Currently, in another pilot, nursing faculty teach alongside a physician colleague during weekly 2-hour small group sessions to mentor first-year medical students role modeling IP collaboration in teaching critical foundational skills, such as communication, professionalism, history taking, discussing difficult and sensitive issues, promoting healthy behaviors, and helping patients make behavior change.

The exemplars in this section presented selected examples of sustained, current, and future IP initiatives from a variety of institutions that are overcoming the many barriers and challenges to IPE. There are many IP initiatives occurring throughout the country, many of which have not been communicated in the literature or at conferences. Those discussed are representative of efforts from throughout the country and selected to show the wide diversity of types of and approaches to IP initiatives as examples for accelerated nursing programs seeking to begin or expand their IP efforts.

CONCLUSION AND FUTURE FOR IPE

Accelerated nursing programs can use interprofessional learning to facilitate realistic professional and practice experiences that will prepare students for their future practice careers. The advantage of IPE for professional relationship building and mutual understanding and respect should improve the care environment, professional satisfaction, and ultimately patient outcomes. Programs on the cutting edge of health professions educational reform need to emphasize to students educated in workable models of IPE that they are pioneers and may face the tremendous challenges associated with the transition to new ways of teaching, learning, and practicing. We are educating and practicing in a time where there are primary care shortages, faculty shortages, and multiple generations of care givers currently practicing, many of whom carry generational biases toward the current work environment and educational system. Graduates and faculty need to be prepared to transition our care delivery model, considering the professional practice environment in which we care for patients who need to navigate complex adaptive health care systems. Patient-centered care provided by teams is the best way to ensure the best outcomes for our patients. Right now, we need to create the plan to address the compelling case put forth by IOM, Carnegie, Josiah Macy, Jr. Foundation, and other interprofessional advocates. The future lies in the present with those faculties, practitioners, and students whom we are currently educating. The time has come for accelerated nursing programs, in partnership with other health professions, to embrace change and partner to prepare contemporary practitioners who are lifelong learners and will ultimately influence future care delivery innovations and ensure the best outcomes for patients and populations.

REFERENCES

American Association of Colleges of Nursing. (1996). Position Statement: Inter disciplinary Education and Practice. *Journal of Professional Nursing, 12*(2), 119–123.

American Association of Colleges of Nursing. (2006). *The essentials of doctoral education for advanced nursing practice.* Retrieved from http://www.aacn.nche. edu/DNP/pdf/Essentials.pdf

American Association of Colleges of Nursing. (2007). *White Paper on the role of the clinical nurse leader.* Retrieved from http://www.aacn.nche.edu/Publications/ WhitePapers/ClinicalNurseLeader.htm

American Association of Colleges of Nursing. (2010a). *Fact Sheet: Accelerated baccalaureate and master's degrees in nursing.* Retrieved from http://www.aacn.nche.edu/publications

American Association of Colleges of Nursing. (2010b). *Issue Bulletin: Accelerated programs: The fast-track to careers in nursing.* Retrieved from http://www.aacn.nche.edu/publications/issues/aug02.htm

American Association of Colleges of Nursing, American Nurses Association, American Organization of Nurse Executives. (2010). *Joint statement from the tri-council for nursing on recent registered nurse supply and demand projections.* Retrieved from http://www.nursingworld.org/MainMenuCategories/HealthcareandPolicyIssues/HealthSystemReform/Registered-Nurse-Supply-and-Demand-Projections.aspx

American Association of Colleges of Nursing & Association of American Medical Colleges. (2010). *Lifelong learning in medicine and nursing final conference report.* Funded by Josiah Macy Foundation. Retrieved http://www.aacn.nche.edu/Education/pdf/MacyReport.pdf

Association of American Medical Colleges. (1995). *Taking charge of the future: The strategic plan for the Association of American Medical Colleges.* Washington, DC: AAMC.

Atkins, J. M., & Walsh, R. S. (1997). Developing shared learning in multiprofessional health care education; for whose benefit? *Nurse Education Today, 17,* 319–324.

Baker, D. P., Gustafson, S., Beaubien, J., Salas, E., & Barach, P. (2005). *Medical teamwork and patient safety: The evidence-based relation: Literature review.* AHRQ Publication No. 05-0053, Rockville, MD: Agency for Healthcare Research and Quality. Retrieved from http://www.ahrq.gov/qual/medteam/

Barr, H. (1998). Competent to collaborate: Towards a competency-based model for interprofessional education. *Journal of Interprofessional Care, 12*(2), 181–187.

Barrington, D., Rodger, M., Gray, L., Jones, B., Langridge, M., & Marriott, R. (1998). Student evaluation of an interactive multi-disciplinary clinical learning model. *Medical Teacher, 20,* 530–535.

Beal, J. (2007). Guest editorial: Accelerated baccalaureate programs: What we know and what we need to know: Setting a research agenda. *Journal of Nursing Education, 46*(9), 387–388.

Benner, P. (2011). Keynote address at the AACN Doctoral Conference, San Diego, CA, 1/27/2011.

Benner, P., Sutphen, M., Leonard, V., & Day, L. (2010). *Educating nurses: A call for radical transformation. The Carnegie Foundation for the Advancement of Teaching.* San Francisco: Jossey-Bass.

Centre for the Advancement of Interprofessional Education. (2002). *Defining IPE: Interprofessional education.* Retrieved from http://www.caipe.org.uk/about-us/defining-ipe/

Chow, M. (2011). In Committee on the Robert Wood Johnson Foundation Initiative on the Future of Nursing, at the Institute of Medicine; Institute of Medicine. *The future of nursing: Leading change, advancing health* (p. 317). Washington, DC: National Academies Press.

Cooke, M., Irby, D. M., & O'Brien, B. C. (2010). *Educating physicians: A call for reform of medical school and residency. The Carnegie Foundation for the Advancement of Teaching.* San Francisco: Jossey-Bass.

Cooper, H., Carlisle, C., Gibbs, T., & Watkins, C. (2001). Developing an evidence base for interdisciplinary learning: A systematic review. *Journal of Advanced Nursing, 35*(2), 228–237.

Cronenwett, L., & Dzau, V. J. (2010). *Who will provide primary care and how will they be trained?* Josiah Macy, Jr. Foundation. Retrieved from www.josiahmacyfoundation.org

Giltell, J. H. (2002). Coordinating mechanisms in care provider groups: Relational coordination as a mediator and input uncertainty as a moderator of performance effects. *Management Science 48*(11), 1408–1426.

Harris, D. L., Starnaman, S. M., Henry, R. C., & Bland, C. J. (1998) Multidisciplinary education outcomes of the W. K. Kellogg community partnerships and health professions education initiative. *Academic Medicine, 73*, S13–S15.

Institute of Medicine. (2000). *To err is human: Building a safer health system.* Washington, DC: The National Academy Press.

Institute of Medicine. (2001). *Crossing the quality chasm.* Washington, DC: The National Academy Press.

Institute of Medicine. (2003). *Health professions education: A bridge to quality.* Washington, DC: The National Academy Press.

Institute of Medicine. (2010 release published 2011). *The future of nursing: Leading change, advancing health.* Washington, DC: The National Academies Press.

Interprofessional Education Collaborative (IPEC) Expert Panel. (2011a). *Core competencies for interprofessional collaborative practice: Report of an expert panel.* Washington, DC: Interprofessional Education Collaborative.

Interprofessional Education Collaborative (IPEC). (2011b). *Team-based competencies: Building a shared foundation for education and clinical practice.* Conference Proceedings: Washington, DC: Interprofessional Education Collaborative.

Josiah Macy Foundation. (2010 Annual Report). *Preparing health professionals for a changing healthcare system.* Retrieved from www.macyfoundation.org

Josiah Macy Foundation Conference Summary. (June 2010). *Educating nurses and physicians: Toward new horizons advancing inter-professional education in Academic Health Centers.* Palo Alto, CA: Author.

Josiah Macy Foundation Grantees. (2010a). Case Western Reserve Interprofessional Learning Exchange and Development Center (I-LEAD). In Josiah Macy, Jr. Foundation. (Annual Report). *Preparing health professionals for a changing healthcare system* (pp. 16–17, 26–27).

Josiah Macy Foundation Grantees. (2010b). University of Colorado REACH (Realizing Educational Advancement for Collaborative Health). In Josiah Macy, Jr. Foundation. (Annual Report). *Preparing health professionals for a changing healthcare system* (pp. 15–16, 26).

Josiah Macy Foundation Grantees. (2010c). Vanderbilt University Fellowship in Interprofessional Learning. In Josiah Macy, Jr. Foundation. (Annual Report). *Preparing health professionals for a changing healthcare system* (pp. 27–28).

Josiah Macy Foundation Grantees. (2010d). Weill Cornell Medical College and Hunter College Integrating Transdisciplinary Education at Cornell Hunter. In Josiah Macy, Jr. Foundation. (Annual Report). *Preparing health professionals for a changing healthcare system* (p. 17).

Luecht, R. M., Madsen, M. K., Taugher, M. P., & Petterson, B. J. (Spring, 1990). Assessing professional perceptions: Design and validation of an interdisciplinary education perception scale. *Journal of Allied Health, 19*(2), 181–191.

Martin, A., Lassman, D., Whittle, L., & Catlin, A. (January 2011). Recession contributes to slowest annual rate of increase in health spending in five decades. *Health Affairs, 30,* 111–122. doi:10.1377/hlthaff.2010.1032.

The Massachusetts Nursing Initiative. (August 2010). *Nurse of the future nursing core competencies.* Retrieved from http://www.mass.edu/currentinit/documents/NursingCoreCompetencies.pdf

McFadyen, A. K., Webster, V., Strachan, K., Figgins, E., Brown, H., & McKechnie, J. (2005). The readiness for interprofessional learning scale: A possible more stable sub-scale model for the original version of RIPLS. *Journal of Interprofessional Care, 19*(6), 595–603.

Miller, B. M., Moore, D. E., Stead, W. W., & Balser, J. R. (2010). Beyond Flexner: A new model for continuous learning in the health professions. *Academic Medicine, 85*(2), 266–272.

Morison, S., Johnston, J., & Stevenson, M. (2010). Preparing students for interprofessional practice: Exploring the intra-personal dimension. *Journal of Interprofessional Care, 24*(4), 412–421.

Parsell, G., & Bligh, J. (1999). The development of a questionnaire to assess the readiness for health care students for interprofessional learning (RIPLS). *Medical Education, 33,* 95–100.

Quality and Safety Education for Nurses (QSEN). (2011). *Quality and Safety Competencies Phase III.* Retrieved from: http://www.qsen.org/about_qsen.php

Reeves, S., Zwarenstein, M., Goldman, J., Barr, H., Freeth, D., Hammick, M. et al. (2009). Interprofessional education: Effects on professional practice and health care outcomes (Review) The Cochrane Collaboration: John Wiley & Sons.

Sarani, B., Sonnad, S., Bergey, M. R., Phillips, J., Fitzpatrick, M. K., Chalian, A. A. et al. (2009). Resident and RN perceptions of the impact of a medical emergency team on education and patient safety in an academic medical center. *Critical Care Medicine, 37*(12), 3091–3096.

Szasz, G. (1969). Interprofessional education in the health sciences. *Milbank Memorial Fund Quarterly, 47,* 449–475.

Thannhauser, J., Russell-Mayhew, S., & Scott, C. (2010). Measures of interprofessional education and collaboration. *Journal of Interprofessional Care, 24*(4), 336–349.

Zwarenstein, M., Goldman, J., & Reeves, S. (2009). Interprofessional collaboration: Effects of practice-based interventions on professional practice and healthcare outcomes (Review). The Cochrane Collaboration: John Wiley & Sons.

Chapter 13

The Growth of Accelerated BSN and MSN Programs in the United States: A National Perspective

Di Fang, Geraldine Polly Bednash, and
Vernell P. DeWitty

*A*ccelerated (or second-degree) baccalaureate and master's programs were designed by nursing schools as an innovative approach to increase schools' education capacities and to meet growing needs of non-nursing college graduates for switching to a nursing career. Having a baccalaureate degree already, these students tend to be more mature, self-motivated, and able to complete their baccalaureate nursing education faster than regular entry-level nursing students (Cangelosi & Whitt, 2005; McDonald, 1995; Seldomridge & DiBartolo, 2005). With the proliferation of the programs in the past decade, a number of studies have been conducted to access these programs. Most of them focused on students' demographic characteristics and academic performance, and others analyzed other aspects of the programs such as curricula for accelerated education and challenges that accelerated program face (Cangelosi & Whitt, 2005; Korvick, Wisener, Lofits, & Williamson, 2008; Bentley, 2006; Meyer, Hoover, & Maposa, 2006; Miklancie & Davis, 2005; Suplee & Glasgow, 2008; Youssef & Goodrich, 1996). However, many of them were based on experiences from a small number of programs, which would limit the generalizability of the study findings. To our knowledge, no study has been conducted on the programs at the national level.

In this study, we analyze the historical growth and recent distribution of these programs at the national level. We also estimate the growth rates needed for future expansion of the programs. In addition, we examine the demographic characteristics of the program participants based on a large number of accelerated programs. We hope our findings will provide the nursing education community and policy makers with better knowledge of the trends and features of the programs, and that this will facilitate expansion of accelerated nursing education.

Our analyses are mainly derived from data collected from the Annual Institutional Data System Survey of the American Association of Colleges of Nursing (AACN). The survey collects data on enrollment, graduation, and faculty from all nursing schools offering baccalaureate and graduate programs and has achieved a high response rate consistently. For example, the response rate was between 81% and 88% in 2001–2010. Additional demographic data are obtained from the New Careers in Nursing Scholarship Program founded by Robert Wood Johnson Foundation, which provides scholarship support to students enrolled in accelerated baccalaureate and master's degree nursing programs.

HISTORICAL GROWTH OF ACCELERATED BSN AND MSN PROGRAMS

The first accelerated baccalaureate program for non-nursing college graduates was introduced at St. Louis University in 1971 (Penprase & Koczara, 2009). In 1990, AACN reported data on the number of such programs for the first time, and 31 academic institutions reported having these accelerated programs (see Table 13.1). The number increased by 90% to 59 in 1994.

However, during the remaining years of the 1990s the programs grew much more slowly. No published data on enrollment and graduations of second-degree BSN programs are available for these years; however, given the dramatic downturn in enrollment in entry-level nursing programs during this time period, one can assume that the numbers of individuals enrolled in second-degree programs also declined. In fact, from 1994 to 2000, enrollment in entry-level baccalaureate programs decreased by 25% (from 97,213 in 1994 to 72,986 in 2000), while graduation declined by 12% (from 26,208 in 1994 to 23,102 in 2000).

The up-and-down trend in entry-level baccalaureate education in the 1990s directly reflected the changing nursing labor market. With the expansion of managed care throughout the United States beginning around 1994, demands for RNs, first in hospitals and later in home health, were significantly reduced. As a result, the nursing shortage in

TABLE 13.1 Growth of Second-Degree and Entry-Level BSN Programs, 1990–2010

YEAR	2ND-DEG. BSN PROGRAMS	2ND-DEG. BSN ENROLLMENT	2ND-DEG. BSN GRADUATION	TOTAL ENTRY-LEVEL BSN PROGRAMS	TOTAL ENTRY-LEVEL BSN ENROLLMENT	TOTAL ENTRY-LEVEL BSN GRADUATION	% OF 2ND-DEG. BSN ENROLLMENT IN TOTAL ENTRY-LEVEL BSN ENROLLMENT	% OF 2ND-DEG. BSN GRADUATION IN TOTAL ENTRY-LEVEL BSN GRADUATION
1990	31			392	78,441	17,129		
1991	43			391	75,771	16,663		
1992	52			407	85,013	18,913		
1993	56			389	89,285	20,912		
1994	59			420	97,213	26,208		
1995	56			416	90,746	27,016		
1996	58			429	87,315	28,354		
1997	66			450	85,488	29,287		
1998	69			430	77,679	27,137		
1999	69			450	75,909	25,404		
2000	70			443	72,986	23,102		
2001	84			464	77,958	22,593		
2002	105			487	85,415	23,665		
2003	128	4,794	1,352	480	95,766	23,621	5.0%	5.7%
2004	150	6,090	2,422	499	112,180	27,394	5.4%	8.8%
2005	173	7,829	3,769	509	124,814	31,827	6.3%	11.8%
2006	187	8,493	5,232	529	133,578	37,851	6.4%	13.8%
2007	195	9,938	5,881	551	141,735	41,500	7.0%	14.2%
2008	209	11,018	6,870	565	145,845	45,339	7.6%	15.2%
2009	224	11,930	7,444	587	151,378	47,121	7.9%	15.8%
2010	228	13,605	8,405	608	161,540	51,039	8.4%	16.5%
Growth 2003–10	78%	184%	522%	27%	69%	116%		

Note: Total Entry-level BSN Programs in this table include traditional entry-level BSN programs and second-degree BSN programs.
Data Source: AACN Annual Survey 1990–2010. Reprinted by permission of American Association of Colleges of Nursing.

the early 1990s ended. While employment growth for RNs slowed to less than 2% during 1994–1997, wage growth for RNs fell annually (Buerhaus & Staiger, 1999). There were widespread reports of nursing layoffs due to lack of employment opportunities in hospitals (Shiber, 2003). The limited career opportunities and earnings served as inhibiting factors to students seeking career options and likely were the most important determinant of the declining enrollment in entry-level programs in nursing.

However, by the end of the 20th century, the nation faced a severe nursing shortage again, and demand for professional nursing staff increased significantly, which resulted in increased interests in a nursing career and enrollment in baccalaureate nursing education programs expanded. Between 2000 and 2010, the number of entry-level BSN programs grew by 37% (from 443 to 608), while the number of accelerated BSN programs increased by a stunning 226% (from 70 to 228). In 2003, when AACN reported enrollment and graduation data on second-degree BSN programs for the first time, 4,794 students were enrolled and 1,352 individuals graduated. By 2010, the number of students and graduates of these programs increased by 184% and 522% (to 13,605 and 8,405), respectively. This growth significantly outpaced the growth in entry-level BSN programs (69% for enrollment and 116% for graduation). As a result, the share of second-degree BSN students in total entry-level BSN enrollment increased from 5% to 8.4%, while their share in total graduates grew from 5.7% to 16.5%. The rapid growth in accelerated BSN enrollment and graduations was due to both expansion of existing programs and introduction of new programs.

The number of master's programs for non-nursing college graduates, another type of second-degree nursing programs, was quite small before 1999 (between 9 and 13 per year, see Table 13.2). However, by 2003, when AACN reported enrollment and graduation data on second-degree master's programs for the first time, the number of programs increased to 28, with 2,046 students and 446 graduates. From 2003 to 2010, the number of such programs grew by 125% (to 63), while enrollment and graduation increased by 174% (to 5,600) and 243% (to 1,528), respectively. Again, growth in second-degree master's programs significantly outpaced those in traditional master's programs. Consequently, the share of second-degree master's students in total master's enrollment increased from 5.5% to 6.5%, while their share in total master's graduations grew from 4.4% to 7%.

Based on data from 45 second-degree BSN programs and 12 second-degree MSN programs in 2010, the average length of time to completion was 14.1 months for baccalaureate degrees and 23.8 months for master's degrees (DeWitty, 2011). These programs reported pre-requisite

TABLE 13.2 Growth of Second-Degree Master's Programs, 1990–2010

YEAR	2ND DEG. MASTER'S PROGRAMS	2ND DEG. MASTER'S ENROLLMENT	2ND DEG. MASTER'S GRADUATION	TOTAL MASTER'S PROGRAMS	TOTAL MASTER'S ENROLLMENT	TOTAL MASTER'S GRADUATION	% OF 2ND DEG. MASTER'S ENROLLMENT IN TOTAL MASTER'S ENROLLMENT	% OF 2ND DEG. MASTER'S GRADUATION IN TOTAL MASTER'S GRADUATION
1990	12							
1991	9							
1992	11							
1993	10							
1994	9							
1995	13							
1996	13							
1997	11							
1998	12							
1999	15							
2000	21							
2001	24							
2002	34							
2003	28	2,046	446	359	37,241	10,030	5.5%	4.4%
2004	41	2,666	542	379	42,751	10,730	6.2%	5.1%
2005	46	3,200	674	392	46,444	12,099	6.9%	5.6%
2006	56	3,854	870	418	56,028	13,470	6.9%	6.5%
2007	56	4,303	1,032	429	62,451	15,182	6.9%	6.8%
2008	55	4,577	1,177	444	69,565	17,247	6.6%	6.8%
2009	65	5,385	1,562	468	77,146	19,063	7.0%	8.2%
2010	63	5,600	1,528	485	86,746	21,730	6.5%	7.0%
Growth 2003–10	125%	174%	243%	35%	133%	117%		

Note: Total Master's Programs in this table include traditional master's programs and second-degree master's Programs.
Data Source: AACN Annual Survey 1990–2010. Reprinted by permission of American Association of Colleges of Nursing.

credit hours of 51.4 prior to admission. These required credit hours were in chemistry, microbiology, anatomy and physiology, psychology, nutrition, and statistics. On average, these accelerated programs require students to complete 805 clinical hours before graduation. Based on AACN data of 228 second-degree BSN programs in 2010, 48.2% did not offer curricula via distance education; 42.5% offered distance education for less than 25% of the course work; and the remaining 9.2% offered distance education for more than 25% of the course work. Of 63 second-degree MSN programs in 2010, 12.7% offered distance education for more than 25% of the course work (Fang, Hu, & Bednash, 2011).

GROWTH VARIATIONS OF SECOND-DEGREE BSN AND MSN PROGRAMS BY INSTITUTIONAL CHARACTERISTICS AND REGION

To better understand the growth of accelerated BSN and MSN programs for non-nursing college graduates, we analyze the distributional changes of the programs, comparing them with entry-level BSN programs and traditional master's programs.

We found that the distribution of entry-level BSN programs changed little across institutional and regional categories between 2003 and 2010. While 26% of the programs were affiliated with doctoral universities in 2003 (based on Carnegie Classification), the figure decreased slightly to 24% in 2010. Meanwhile, the percentage for the programs instituted in master's colleges or universities changed little from 48% to 49% (see Table 13.3). In comparison, 45% of second-degree BSN programs were affiliated with doctoral universities in 2003, indicating that such programs were highly concentrated in large research universities in early years of the 2000s. However, the figure decreased significantly to 35% by 2010, while the percentage for the programs in master's colleges or universities increased from 37% to 44%, indicating that more new second-degree BSN programs were introduced in master's institutions than doctoral institutions. The percentage change for institutions in the "Other" category, most of which were classified as medical schools or other health professional schools by Carnegie Classification, also increased from 9% to 14%.

While the distribution of entry-level BSN programs changed little by public or private institution status between 2003 and 2010, the percentage for second-degree BSN programs operated in public institutions increased from 41% to 54%, suggesting new second-degree BSN programs were more likely to be introduced in public schools in those years. While the percentage distribution of entry-level BSN programs located in the North Atlantic Region changed little from 21% to 20%, accelerated BSN programs

TABLE 13.3 Distribution and Enrollment Growth of Second-Degree BSN Programs, 2003–2010

INSTITUTION CHARACTERISTICS	DISTRIBUTION OF ENTRY-LEVEL BSN PROGRAMS IN 2003	DISTRIBUTION OF ENTRY-LEVEL BSN PROGRAMS IN 2010	DISTRIBUTION OF 2ND-DEG. BSN PROGRAMS IN 2003	DISTRIBUTION OF 2ND-DEG. BSN PROGRAMS IN 2010	MEAN ENROLLMENT IN 2ND-DEG. BSN PROGRAMS IN 2003	MEAN ENROLLMENT IN 2ND-DEG. BSN PROGRAMS IN 2010	GROWTH RATE OF MEAN ENROLLMENT IN 2ND-DEG. BSN PROGRAMS 2003–10	DISTRIBUTION OF TOTAL ENROLLMENT IN 2ND-DEG. BSN PROGRAMS IN 2003	DISTRIBUTION OF TOTAL ENROLLMENT IN 2ND-DEG. BSN PROGRAMS IN 2010
Doctoral Universities	26%	24%	45%	35%	50	74	48%	60%	44%
Master's Colleges/Universities	48%	49%	37%	44%	31	45	44%	32%	33%
Baccalaureate Colleges	17%	18%	9%	7%	10	33	223%	2%	4%
Others	10%	9%	9%	14%	26	84	224%	6%	19%
Public	51%	49%	41%	54%	37	51	40%	40%	46%
Private/Secular	15%	15%	31%	20%	47	88	86%	38%	29%
Private/Religious	34%	36%	29%	27%	29	56	96%	22%	25%
North Atlantic	21%	20%	33%	26%	48	70	47%	42%	30%
Midwest	32%	32%	26%	29%	29	48	64%	20%	23%
South	35%	35%	30%	34%	37	57	55%	29%	32%
West	12%	13%	12%	12%	29	76	163%	9%	14%
Total	N = 476	N = 588	N = 128	N = 228	38	60	57%	N = 4,794	N = 13,605

Note: Entry-level BSN programs in this table do not include second-degree BSN programs.
Data Source: AACN Annual Survey 2003–2010. Reprinted by permission of American Association of Colleges of Nursing.

in the same region decreased substantially from 33% to 26%. Meanwhile, the percentage of accelerated BSN programs in Midwest and South regions increased from 26% to 29% and 30% to 34%, respectively. The geographic distribution of second-degree BSN programs was more similar to that of entry-level BSN programs by the end of the 2003–2010 period.

The distributional changes of second-degree BSN programs were also accompanied by growth in individual programs' total enrollment. Between 2003 and 2010, the mean number of students per program in second-degree BSN programs increased by 57% from 38 to 56 nationally. In doctoral institutions, due to a decrease in the portion of BSN programs that were accelerated (from 45% to 35%) and a slower enrollment growth (48%) than the national average of 57%, the portion of total enrollment in these programs decreased from 60% to 44%. The finding seems to indicate a decrease in the portion of students who are in accelerated BSN programs in large research universities. Given a decreased share in total number of programs and a lower growth rate in enrollment, such programs in the North Atlantic region also dropped their share in total enrollment from 42% to 30%. Although the enrollment growth for programs in public institutions (40%) was below the national average, their share in total enrollment still increased from 40% to 46% because of a significant increase in their share in the total number of programs (from 41% to 54%).

Interestingly, the patterns of distributional change and enrollment growth for second-degree MSN programs were quite similar to those for second-degree BSN programs during the same period: For accelerated MSN programs instituted in doctoral universities, their share in the total number of programs decreased from 64% to 51%, and their enrollment growth (15%) was below the national average (22%). Consequently, their share in total enrollment decreased from 70% to 53% (see Table 13.4). For programs located in the North Atlantic region, their share in total enrollment decreased from 37% to 22%, as a result of a decreased contribution to total number of programs (from 36% to 24%) and a slower enrollment growth (12%) than the national average. On the other hand, for programs operated in public institutions, their share in total enrollment increased from 35% to 45%, which was largely resulted from their share increase in the total number of programs (from 46% to 56%).

DEMOGRAPHIC CHARACTERISTICS OF STUDENTS IN SECOND-DEGREE PROGRAMS

Previous studies indicated that with a higher percentage of men, underrepresented minority groups, and non-US residents, second-degree programs had a more diverse student population than traditional programs

TABLE 13.4 Distribution and Enrollment Growth of Second-Degree Master's Programs, 2003–2010

INSTITUTION CHARACTERISTICS	DISTRIBUTION OF TRADITIONAL MASTER'S PROGRAMS IN 2003	DISTRIBUTION OF TRADITIONAL MASTER'S PROGRAMS IN 2010	DISTRIBUTION OF 2ND-DEG. MSN PROGRAMS IN 2003	DISTRIBUTION OF 2ND-DEG. MSN PROGRAMS IN 2010	MEAN ENROLLMENT IN 2ND-DEG. MSN PROGRAMS IN 2003	MEAN ENROLLMENT IN 2ND-DEG. MSN PROGRAMS IN 2010	MEAN ENROLLMENT GROWTH IN 2ND-DEG. MSN PROGRAMS 2003–10	DISTRIBUTION OF TOTAL ENROLLMENT IN 2ND-DEG. MSN PROGRAMS IN 2003	DISTRIBUTION OF TOTAL ENROLLMENT IN 2ND-DEG. MSN PROGRAMS IN 2010
Doctoral Universities	33%	31%	64%	51%	80	92	15%	70%	53%
Master's Col1eges/Lhiversities	53%	51%	18%	33%	47	60	28%	12%	23%
Baccalaureate Col1eges	3%	8%	0%	0%	na	na	na	0%	0%
Others	11%	10%	18%	16%	74	139	88%	18%	25%
Public	53%	52%	46%	56%	55	71	29%	35%	45%
Private/Secular	16%	19%	29%	19%	124	150	21%	49%	32%
Private/religious	31%	29%	25%	25%	49	81	65%	17%	23%
North Atlantic	26%	26%	36%	24%	75	84	12%	37%	22%
Midwest	25%	27%	25%	24%	44	87	98%	15%	23%
South	36%	33%	21%	19%	99	87	–12%	29%	19%
west	13%	14%	18%	33%	78	95	22%	19%	36%
Total	N = 289	N = 484	N = 28	N = 63	73	89	22%	N = 2,046	N = 5,600

Data Source: AACN Annual Survey 2003–2010. Reprinted by permission of American Association of Colleges of Nursing.

(Cangelosi & Whitt, 2005; Stuenkel, Nelson, Malloy, & Cohen, 2011; Suplee & Glasgow, 2008). However, such findings were often based on data from a small number of programs. Based on data from a large number of programs, we compare the race/ethnicity and gender distributions of second-degree BSN and MSN students and graduates with their counterparts in entry-level BSN and traditional MSN programs to determine if these differences are seen in a larger population.

We found that of 6,137 students from 82 second-degree BSN programs, 62.7% were white. In comparison, of total 28,454 students in 82 entry-level BSN programs from the same schools, 69.5% were white (see Table 13.5). However, the percentages for African Americans, Hispanics, Asians, Native Americans, and Pacific Islanders were quite similar between the two types of programs, while the percentage for the "Other" category among second-degree students was higher than that for entry-level BSN students (11.7% vs. 7.6%). Since international students would be included in the "Other" category, the finding seems to indicate a higher presence of non-US residents in second-degree programs. For 3,757 second-degree BSN graduates and 8,487 entry-level BSN graduates from the same 71 schools, the differences in race/ethnicity distributions were even smaller. However, we did find that men had a higher presentation among second-degree students (16.7% vs. 11%) and graduates (15.7% vs. 10.6%) than that for entry-level BSN students and graduates.

There were no clear discrepancies in race/ethnicity distributions between 5,600 second-degree MSN students and 12,469 traditional

TABLE 13.5 Demographic Characteristics of Second-Degree and Entry-Level BSN Students and Graduates from Same Schools

DEMOGRAPHIC CHARACTERISTICS	2ND-DEG. BSN ENROLLMENT IN 2009	ENTRY-LEVEL BSN ENROLLMENT IN 2009	2ND-DEG. BSN GRADUATION IN 2009	ENTRY-LEVEL BSN GRADUATION IN 2009
Number of Programs	82	82	71	71
Number of Students	6,137	28,454	3,757	8,487
% White	62.7%	69.5%	65.7%	68.3%
% African American	10.7%	9.9%	9.4%	9.6%
% Hispanic	5.8%	5.5%	6.1%	5.9%
% Asian	8.0%	6.4%	7.9%	6.4%
% Pacific Islander	0.6%	0.4%	0.5%	0.3%
% Native	0.5%	0.7%	0.4%	0.7%
% Other	11.7%	7.6%	10.0%	8.8%
% Male	16.7%	11.0%	15.7%	10.6%

Data Source: Entry-Level BSN data were collected by AACN Annual Survey 2009. Second-degree BSN data were obtained from Robert Wood Johnson Foundation's New Careers in Nursing Scholarship Program.

master's students, and between 1,528 second-degree MSN graduates and 3,637 traditional master's graduates, all from the same 63 schools (see Table 13.6). Although the percentage of men among second-degree master's students and graduates was consistently higher than that for their counterparts in traditional master's programs, the magnitude of the difference was only about 3%.

In brief, we did not find that students and graduates in second-degree BSN or MSN programs were more diverse than their counterparts in entry-level BSN or traditional MSN programs. Although men consistently had a higher presentation in second-degree programs than in traditional programs, the difference at the master's level is not substantial.

FUTURE GROWTH OF SECOND-DEGREE BSN PROGRAMS

As we reported above, second-degree BSN programs experienced a tremendous growth in the past decade. What is the likelihood that the growth will continue in the future? We address this question in this study.

Table 13.1 shows that there were 128 second-degree BSN programs with 4,794 students in 2003. By 2010, the number of programs increased to 228 with 13,605 students. Further analyses show that of the 128 programs initiated in 2003, 24 were closed in a later year, while 104 remained active by 2010. Meanwhile, 124 new programs were started between

TABLE 13.6 Demographic Characteristics of Second-Degree and Traditional Master's Students from Same Schools

DEMOGRAPHIC CHARACTERISTICS	2ND-DEG. MSN ENROLLMENT IN 2010	TRADITIONAL MSN ENROLLMENT IN 2010	2ND-DEG. MSN GRADUATION IN 2010	TRADITIONAL MSN GRADUATION IN 2010
Number of Programs	63	63	63	63
Number of Students	5,600	12,469	1,528	3,637
% White	60.5%	68.0%	64.9%	64.0%
% African American	6.1%	8.7%	4.9%	8.3%
% Hispanic	5.6%	3.9%	4.6%	3.3%
% Asian	12.1%	7.8%	12.4%	7.5%
% Pacific Islander	0.4%	0.4%	0.3%	0.4%
% Native	0.5%	0.7%	0.5%	0.7%
% Non-US Resident	1.1%	1.8%	1.4%	1.3%
% Other	13.7%	8.7%	11.0%	14.5%
% Male	12.8%	10.2%	12.0%	9.3%

Data Source: AACN Annual Survey 2010. Reprinted by permission of American Association of Colleges of Nursing.

2003 and 2010. Of the 13,605 students in 2010, 7,323 (53.8%) came from the 104 remaining programs, and the other 6,282 students (46.2%) were from the 124 newly introduced programs. During this period, total enrollment in the 104 remaining programs grew by 78% (from 4,112 to 7,323), with an annual growth rate of 11.1% (78%/7).

Given the significant contribution of new programs to total enrollment in accelerated baccalaureate programs, we need to have a better knowledge of numbers of new programs planned and introduced per year. A total of 49 schools reported program planning for a second-degree BSN program in 2003. However, we found that more than a half of them also reported similar plans in previous years, and only 22 (45%) reported such plans for the first time (see Table 13.7). Of all programs planned between 2003 and 2010, 134 (46%) were such new programs. Of the 121 new programs planned between 2003 and 2009, 58 were introduced by 2010. (Note for the 13 new programs planned in 2010, we do not have information regarding their program introducing status.) In addition, we found that there were 54 schools that did not report program planning but introduced a program between 2003 and 2010. Accordingly, we estimated the total number of new programs planned is 188 (134 + 54) during this period, averaging 23.5 new programs planned per year. In addition to the 112 (58 + 54) newly introduced programs mentioned above, there were another 12 schools that planned a program prior to 2003 and introduced it in 2003 or a later year. As a whole, there were a total of 124 new programs (58 + 54 + 12) introduced between 2003 and 2010, averaging 15.5 programs introduced per year.

Planning for new programs is often directly related to employment opportunities in nursing and the perceived desirability of a nursing career in the potential student population. Thus, accelerated nursing programs can be a powerful attractor to students seeking a career change, provided the employment options are robust. Based on a recent AACN

TABLE 13.7 Second-Degree BSN Programs Planned and Opened, 2008–2010

	2003	2004	2005	2006	2007	2008	2009	2010	TOTAL
Number of programs planned	49	46	39	36	32	26	33	31	292
Number of new programs opened	22	21	16	13	14	15	20	13	134
% as programs planned for the first time	45%	43%	35%	33%	39%	47%	77%	39%	46%

Data Source: AACN Annual Survey 2002–2010. Reprinted by permission of American Association of Colleges of Nursing.

survey on employment of new graduates from entry-level BSN and MSN programs in 393 nursing schools (American Association of Colleges of Nursing, 2010), we found that 89% of new graduates had job offers within 4–6 months after graduation. Thus, despite the current recession, nursing graduates continue to see robust employment options and nursing continues as one of a limited bright spots in the job market. This seems to indicate that the demand for accelerated nursing education among college graduates with a non-nursing degree is likely to continue. If we want to maintain a similar growth rate in total enrollment for second-degree BSN education that was experienced in 2003–2010, for existing second-degree BSN programs, their enrollment needs to continue to grow at 11.1% annually. In addition, roughly 25 new programs need to be planned, and of them, 16 need to be introduced per year, based on our analyses above.

Why have some planned programs failed to be introduced? We do not have data to answer this question directly. However, we found there are some differences in institutional characteristics between the programs that were introduced successfully and programs that were planned but failed to be introduced. Only 7% of programs introduced successfully were instituted in baccalaureate colleges. In comparison, 24% of planned programs that failed to be introduced were from those colleges (see Table 13.8). While 62% of programs were introduced successfully were from public institutions, the figure is 52% for programs failed to be introduced. On the other hand, 35% of planned programs that failed to be introduced were from private/religious institutions, and the figure is 23% for successfully introduced programs. In brief, programs introduced

TABLE 13.8 Distribution of Planned Second-Degree BSN Programs by Program Opening Status

INSTITUTION CHARACTERISTICS	NEW PROGRAM OPENED, 2003–2010	PLANNED PROGRAMS FAILED TO OPEN, 2003–2010
Doctoral Universities	27%	17%
Master's Colleges/Universities	49%	51%
Baccalaureate Colleges	7%	24%
Others	17%	8%
Public	62%	52%
Private/Secular	15%	13%
Private/Religious	23%	35%
Total	$N = 124$	$N = 63$

Data Source: AACN Annual Survey 2002–2010. Reprinted by permission of American Association of Colleges of Nursing.

successfully were more likely to be instituted in larger public universities than programs that failed to be introduced, which were more likely to be planned by smaller private/religious colleges.

SUMMARY AND DISCUSSION

In this study, we analyze the historical growth and current distributions of second-degree BSN and MSN programs based on national-level data. We also estimate the growth rates needed for continuing the expansion of these programs in the near future. We have the following findings:

First, second-degree BSN and MSN programs grew faster than entry-level BSN and traditional master's programs in terms of enrollment and graduation in the past decade. As a result, their share in enrollment and graduation in total entry-level baccalaureate programs and master's programs increased. Second, new second-degree BSN and MSN programs were more likely to be introduced in master's institutions and public schools as the share of programs in these types of institutions grew over the past decade. Thirdly, consistent with findings from previous studies, we found that the proportion of male students, and likely international students, in second-degree programs was higher than that in entry-level BSN and traditional master's programs. However, we did not find that second-degree students were more diverse than students from traditional programs in terms of race/ethnicity composition. Finally, we found that almost half of enrollment growth in second-degree BSN programs between 2003 and 2010 was contributed by programs introduced during this time period. Based on our estimates, to maintain a growth rate similar to that in the 2003–2010 period, existing programs need to maintain an 11.1% growth rate annually, while roughly 25 new programs need to be planned, and of them, 16 need to be introduced. In addition, we found that for planned programs that failed to be introduced, they were more likely than programs that were introduced successfully to be instituted in smaller private/religious institutions. We hope these findings will enhance the planning capacity of the nursing education community for second-degree programs.

Our analyses are based on national data collected in the AACN Annual Survey of Baccalaureate and Graduate Programs in Nursing. Given the high response rate (81–88% in 2001–2010), we believe our findings show the national patterns and trends in accelerated nursing education. Although part of our data, such as demographic information for second-degree BSN programs and average length of time to program completion for second-degree programs, are not collected from a national representative survey, given the large number of programs and students included, we believe that the data are still informative.

To continue the expansion of accelerated nursing education, we also need to have a better knowledge of the challenges encountered by existing programs. In this regard, the following lessons learned by 63 second-degree BSN and MSN programs, which participated in the New Career in Nursing Scholarship Program funded by Robert Wood Johnson Foundation, for which two of our coauthors (Bednash & DeWitty) are the Director and Deputy Director, would be useful:

(1) Psychological supports: Although accelerated degree students are mature with past careers and life experiences, the challenges these students experienced are still significant. Using student mentors is found to be successful; however, this must be a guided process where each student is either a mentee or mentor. (2) Program preparation: Many students know that the program is rigorous, but do not anticipate how challenging the pace can be. Having a preparatory experience helps students build the confidence and skills needed to manage the demands of the program. (3) Student selection: In addition to standardized entrance exams and GPA assessments, a written essay and interview as part of the admission assessment is effective. (4) Faculty involvement: When faculty closely monitor the progress of each student, they are able to help students resolve challenges that students face in the course of their study (DeWitty, 2011).

Clearly, accelerated nursing programs for career changers are tapping a market of students with a strong interest in nursing. Moreover, the career and employment options for these students remain strong despite the economic downturn. This would seem to indicate that these programs will continue to maintain strong enrollment, continue to expand in size and numbers, and have great attractiveness to the institutions that implement these programs. One must caution the reader, however, that the nuances of economics in higher education and our nation will have direct and continuing effects on the growth potential in these programs. They, however, remain a strong indication of the creative and flexible nature of nursing education in baccalaureate and graduate degree granting institutions.

REFERENCES

American Association of Colleges of Nursing. (2010). Employment of new nurse graduates from entry-level baccalaureate programs. *Research Brief*, November. Retrieved from http://www.aacn.nche.edu/IDS/pdf/ResBriefEmpl.pdf

Bentley, R. (2006). Comparison of traditional and accelerated baccalaureate nursing graduates. *Nurse Educator, 31*(2), 79–83.

Buerhaus, P. I., & Staiger, D. O. (1999). Trouble in the nurse labor market? Recent trends and future outlook. *Health Affairs, 18*(1), 214–222.

Cangelosi, P. R., & Whitt, K. J. (2005). Accelerated nursing programs: What do we know? *Nursing Education Perspectives, 26*(2), 113–116.

DeWitty, V. (2011). *Report on new careers in nursing scholarship program of Robert Wood Johnson Foundation* (unpublished data). Washington, DC: American Association of Colleges of Nursing.

Fang, D., Hu, E., & Bednash, G. D. (2011). *2010–2011 Enrollment and Graduations in Baccalaureate and Graduate Programs in Nursing, Table 13.4b*. Washington, DC: American Association of Colleges of Nursing.

Korvick, L. M., Wisener, L. K., Loftis, L. A., & Williamson, M. L. (2008). Comparing the academic performance of students in traditional and second-degree baccalaureate programs. *Journal of Nursing Education, 47*(3), 139–141.

McDonald, W. K. (1995). Comparison of performance of students in an accelerated baccalaureate nursing program for college graduates and a traditional nursing program. *Journal of Nursing Education, 34*(3), 123–127.

Meyer, G. A., Hoover, K. G., & Maposa, S. (2006). A profile of accelerated BSN graduates, 2004. *Journal of Nursing Education, 45*(8), 324–327.

Miklancie, M., & Davis, T. (2005). The second-degree accelerated program as an innovative educational strategy: New century, new chapter, new challenge. *Nursing Education Perspectives, 26*(5), 291–293.

Penprase, B., & Koczara, S. (2009). Understanding the experiences of accelerated second-degree nursing students and graduates: A review of literature. *Journal of Continuing Education in Nursing, 40*(2), 74–78.

Seldomridge, L. A., & DiBartolo, M. C. (2005). A profile of accelerated second bachelor's degree nursing students. *Nurse Educator, 30*(2), 65–68.

Shiber, S. (2003). A nursing education model for second-degree students. *Nursing Education Perspectives, 24*(3), 135–138.

Stuenkel, D., Nelson, D., Malloy, S., & Cohen, J. (2011). Challenges, changes, and collaboration: Evaluation of an accelerated BSN program. *Nurse Educator, 36*(2), 70–75.

Suplee, P., & Glasgow, M. (2008). Curriculum innovation in an accelerated BSN program: The ACE model. *International Journal of Nursing Education Scholarship, 5*(1), 1–13.

Youssef, F. A., & Goodrich, N. (1996). Accelerated versus traditional nursing students: A comparison of stress, critical thinking ability and performance. *International Journal of Nursing Studies, 33*(1), 76–82.

Index